SOMATIC YOGA

Low-Impact Exercises to Reduce Belly Fat and Release Stress in Just 10 Minutes per Day | 28-Day Plan for Beginners

Merton Corey

Copyright:

© 2024 Merton Corey. All rights reserved. No part of this publication may be reproduced, distributed, or transmitted in any form or by any means, including photocopying, recording, or other electronic or mechanical methods, without the prior written permission of the publisher, except in the case of brief quotations embodied in critical reviews and certain other noncommercial uses permitted by copyright law.

Disclaimer:

The information provided in this book is intended for general informational and educational purposes only. The author is not a licensed medical professional, and the content in this book should not be considered a substitute for professional medical advice, diagnosis, or treatment. Always seek the advice of your physician or qualified healthcare provider before beginning any fitness program or making significant changes to your diet or exercise routine.

The author and publisher have made reasonable efforts to ensure that the information presented in this book is accurate and reliable at the time of publication. However, they do not warrant the completeness, reliability, or accuracy of this information. The author and publisher disclaim any liability for any adverse effects or consequences resulting from the use of the information contained herein, either directly or indirectly.

By reading this book, you acknowledge and agree that you are solely responsible for any actions you take based on the information provided, and you release the author and the publisher from any liability for any damages or injuries, whether direct or indirect, that may result.

TABLE OF CONTENTS

INTRODUCTION..4
   WHY DOING SOMATIC YOGA?.. 5
   5 TIPS TO STAY MOTIVATED.. 6
HOW TO READ THE BOOK TO GET THE BEST OUT OF IT..............7
EXERCISES...9
   FLOATED CRAWLING... 9
   SEATED WINDSHIELD WIPERS... 11
   ROLLING PATTERN.. 13
   BRUSHING BODY DOWN... 15
   OPEN HEART..17
   KNEE GRAB LYING... 19
   KNEE GRAB SEATED..21
   GROIN RELEASE.. 23
   SOMATIC HIP MOVEMENT... 25
   PUSH OUT IN FRONT... 27
   SKIING..29
   SOMATIC SHAKING...31
   HIP ROCKING ON STOMACH... 33
   LATERAL LUNGE AND REACH... 35
   FAWN.. 37
   DOWNWARD DOG... 39
   ROBOT.. 41
   PIGEON POSE... 43
   BREATHING CIRCLE... 45
   PUSH WALL..47
   STOMP YOUR HEELS... 49
   RUN SHAKE... 51
   STAND ROCK SIDE TO SIDE.. 53
   STAND ROCK BACK AND FORTH.. 55
   FRONTAL RELEASE LUNGE... 57
28-DAY PLAN.. 59
CONCLUSION.. 75

INTRODUCTION

In our hectic and demanding lifestyles we often feel anxious, tense, and overwhelmed. The habitual nature of these negative emotions can make it difficult to break free, and unfortunately, not enough is often done to balance them with positive feelings like joy, energy, mindfulness, and fulfillment.

Somatic yoga aims to help you effectively manage emotional challenges. These exercises are extremely useful for resetting the nervous system and promoting overall well-being. Somatic workouts offer an option to release the negativity that is trapped in our bodies, allowing us to permanently expel these unsettling sensations. These routines will serve you as a therapeutic outlet for people to confront and relieve anxiety, worry, and tension. They will promote a profound sense of relaxation and inner balance by promoting a mind-body connection.

The fact that somatic yoga can be done anywhere makes it a practice particularly accessible and beneficial. All that is required is a mat and a small amount of space. Also, because of their adaptability, these exercises can be incorporated into your daily routine, whether at home, at the office, or even during a break outside.

The main goal of the book is to help you lose weight. Indeed, a key objective of the book is to carefully select exercises and formulate a 28-day plan focused on enhancing weight loss and improved physical well-being. By following the book, you'll witness noticeable improvements in your physical shape (Diet is as well as important as exercise, so make sure to keep that on track too!)

WHY DOING SOMATIC YOGA?

- **Reset nervous system**

Somatic yoga is a fantastic practice for resetting your nervous system, helping you connect with your feelings. When you focus on your breath and stay present during the exercises, it enhances your well-being. Regular practice of these exercises can effectively release the tension and stress you may be carrying, leaving you feeling better overall.

- **Lose weight**

These exercises are excellent for burning calories and losing weight. While these exercises may not be extremely demanding compared to other types, they still provide effective benefits for weight loss.

Following a healthy diet and being in a caloric deficit is also tremendously important for weight loss, as already mentioned.

- **"Release Valve" of your day**

It is the moment of the day to let go of accumulated stress. It is a moment that, once finished, will leave you feeling refreshed.
Turn off your phone and all the other distractions, and enjoy the practice!

- **Cultivate awareness**

Somatic exercises increase body awareness and promote a sense of presence, building the link between your mind and body. Each exercise demands your attention to how you move your body, promoting profound calmness, which strengthens the mind-body connection even more.

- **Better physical health.**

You can also expect to feel the benefits after a few days of consistent exercise, particularly in the lower back, knee, and hip region. This will relieve general tightness and give you a feeling of health and higher levels of energy.

5 TIPS TO STAY MOTIVATED

- **Have an accountability partner**

Keeping consistent will be much easier if you share your journey with someone, and it's even better if you perform these exercises together.

- **Imagine who you will be at the end of the 28 days**

Visualize your goal in your mind. What does your dream body look like? How do you want to feel? Imagine experiencing those feelings and use them as motivation, knowing that with consistency, you will achieve them.

- **Remember why you started**

When you lose motivation or feel "too busy," remember why you started. Write it down if needed, as a reminder, to provide you with the strength to persevere. Doing this from the very beginning will help. So the moment in which you'll lose some motivation (eventually it'll happen to anyone) you can quickly refocus by reminding yourself why you started.

- **Keep a journal**

Write down how you feel after each session and document how the session went in a journal. This will help you track your progress and see how far you have come over time. After the 28-days you will be glad to have documented your sensations day by day.

- **Read "WHY DOING SOMATIC YOGA?"**

The previous chapter outlines the benefits that these workouts offer, emphasizing consistency and motivation. Additionally, following the exercise explanations, there is an introductory page for the 28-day plan, which can also be perused for additional motivation.

HOW TO READ THE BOOK TO GET THE BEST OUT OF IT

It is recommended that you first review the exercises in order to comprehend their patterns and techniques. Familiarizing yourself with them will give you an idea of what to expect to do. After that, go through the 28-Day Plan and begin doing the workouts on a daily basis.

This book is divided into two sections: Exercise and the 28-Day Plan.

The exercises include step-by-step photos and full instructions on how to complete each one. While executing the exercises, remember to exhale through your mouth and inhale through your nose. At the end of each exercise, the duration or the number of repetitions of specific positions are not shown. Every day, you will be expected to execute exercises that differ from those performed the previous day, and the plan is designed to gradually increase the number of sets and repetitions as you develop. Therefore, this information can be found in the section that follows.

The 28-day training plan will be shown in the final section. Follow the daily plan regularly, don't skip workouts, maintain consistency, and stick to it. The outcomes are promised!

Hey! Before we start with the Somatic Yoga and the 28-Day Plan

If you have any doubts, questions or simply you like to give a feedback, feel free to send an email at **mertoncoreyfitness@gmail.com**

I'll be happy to help you maximize your results!

EXERCISES

FLOATED CRAWLING

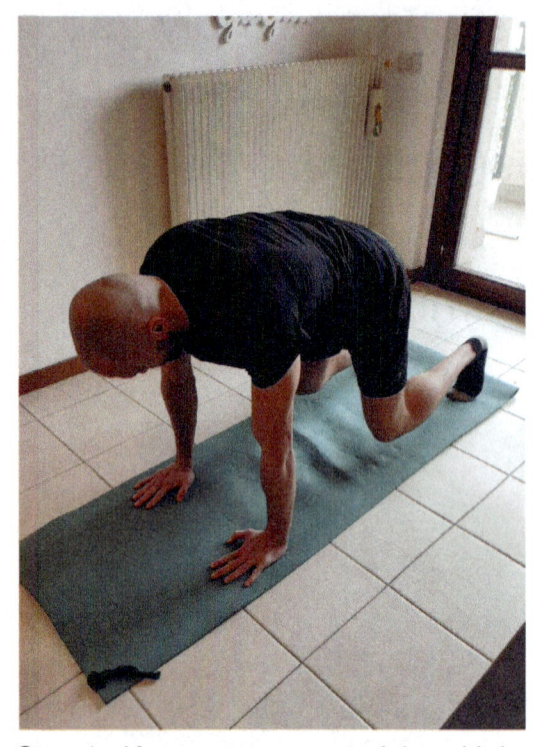

Step 1 - Keep your arms straight, with hands and toes on the mat and lift your knees off the floor.

Step 2 - Bring your buttocks against your heels while keeping your knees lifted. Repeat for the mentioned reps

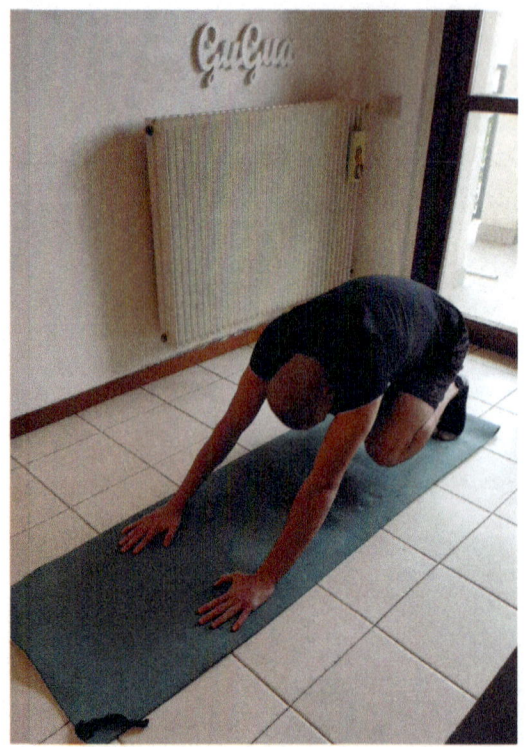

SCAN HERE FOR THE VIDEO TUTORIAL

How to do it:

- Hands on the mat with arms straight and shoulders above them. Keep the core engaged, bend your knees to engage the quads, and keep them elevated - only toes and hands are on the mat. Hold the position for 1 second, while inhaling through your nose.
- Then, exhale and gently bring your buttocks close to your heels to stretch your back keeping your knees elevated and having your arms straight, as shown in Step 2. Hold the position for 1 second.
- Lastly, return to the starting position and perform it for the mentioned repetitions.

Note:

Perform the exercise slowly and maintain control over your body. It requires strength and balance. Exhale deeply via your mouth to let go of any tension, making yourself feel present.

SEATED WINDSHIELD WIPERS

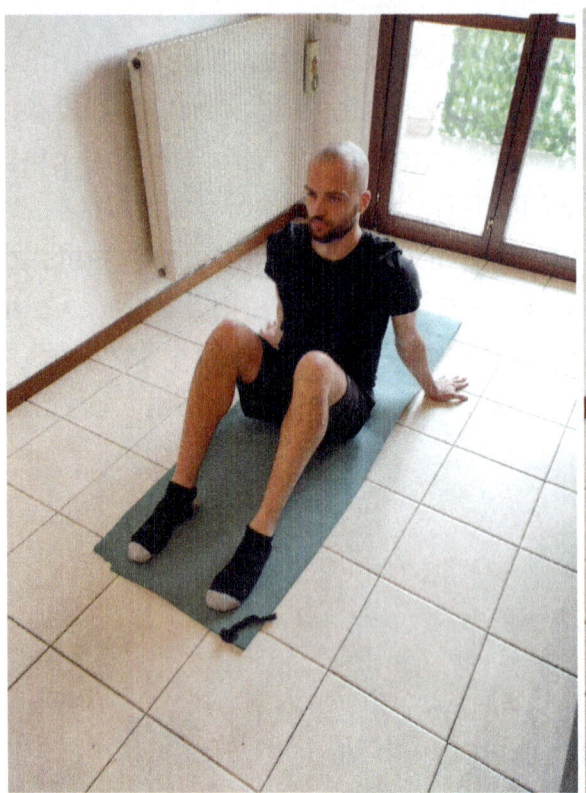

Step 1 - Sit on the mat with hands on the floor, knees bent.

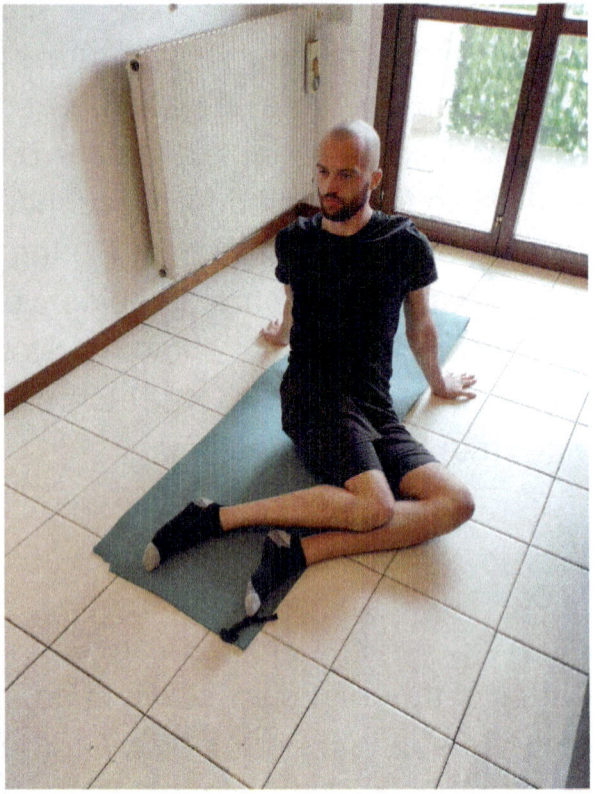

Step 2 - Keep your spine erect while moving your knees to the left side.

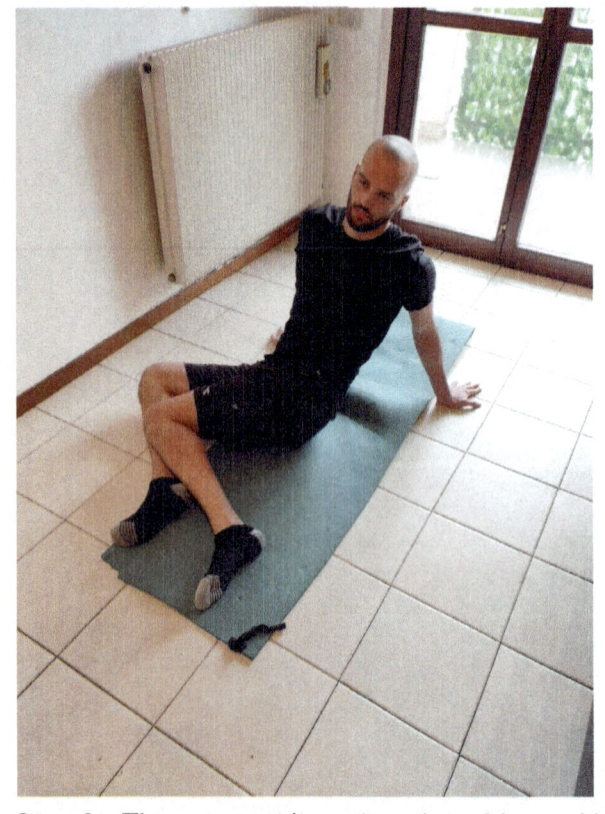

Step 3 - Then, repeat it on the other side, and keep alternating between the sides.

How to do it:

- Sit on the mat with hands on the floor, spine erect, looking forward, knees bent, and feet on the floor.
- Whilst keeping the back straight, move your knees to the left, almost touching the floor. Then, turn them to the other side - this counts as one rep. Keep breathing softly as you perform the movement.
- Repeat for the mentioned reps.

Note:

Be mindful while doing the exercise and focus on moving your hips side to side. Great exercises to release stiffness on your hips, a place where we tend to store considerable amounts of tension.

ROLLING PATTERN

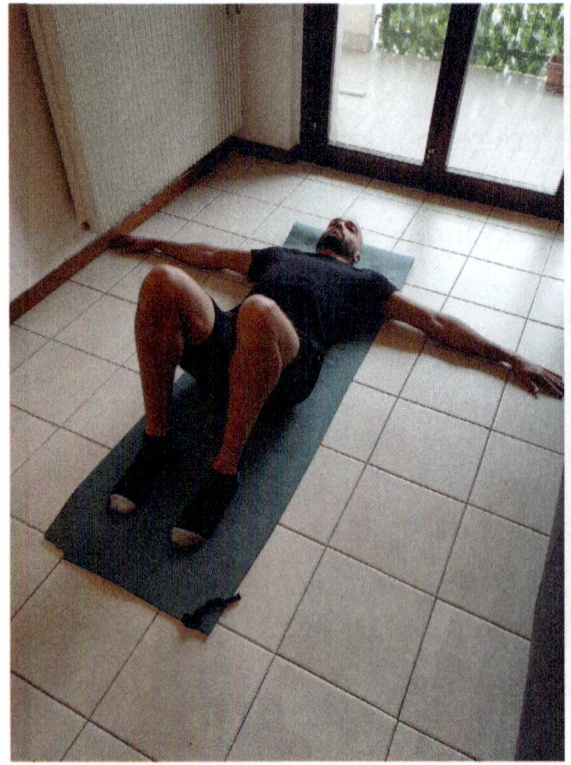

Step 1 - Lie on the mat with knees bent and feet on the floor. Arms open at a 90-degree angle.

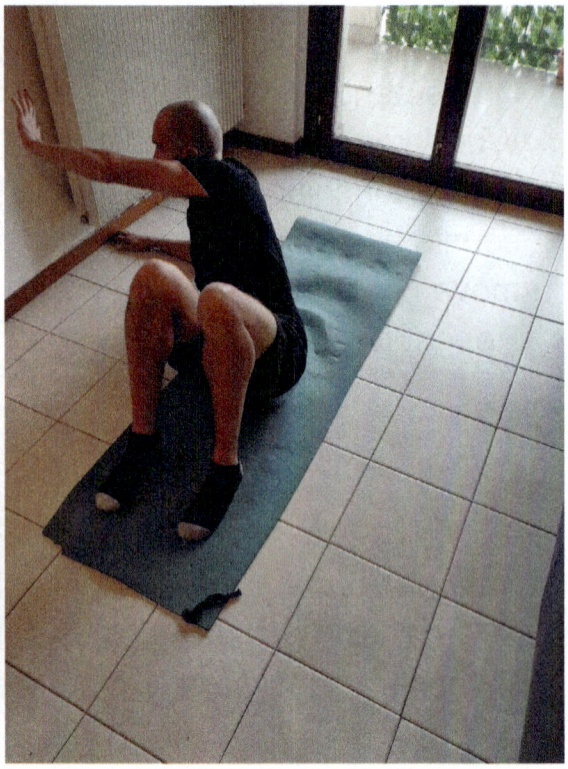

Step 2 - Perform a half sit-up and twist and lift your back by bringing the left arm towards the right side at shoulder height.

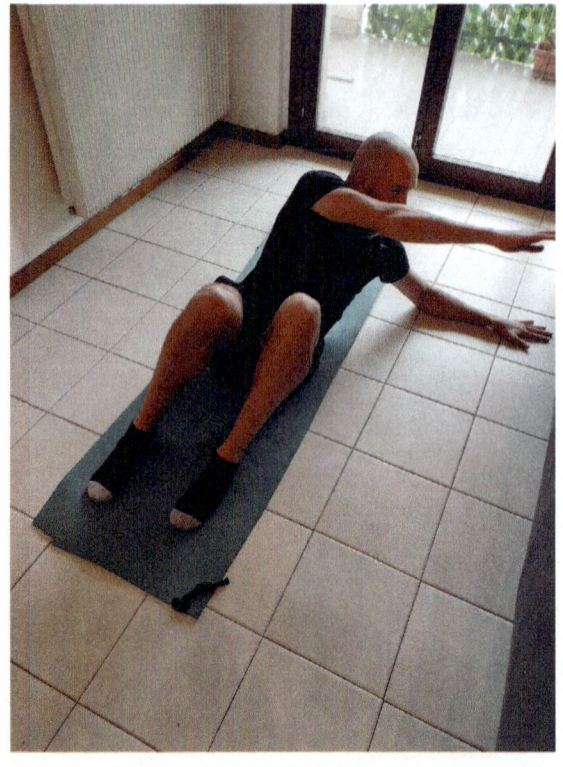

Step 3 - Then, come back to the starting position, and repeat it on the other side.

How to do it:

- Lie on the mat with your back, knees bent, feet on the floor, and arms open on the floor at a 90-degree angle. Keep your neck relaxed, looking up. Be still and relaxed, breathing gently.
- Then, lift your back up, like a crunch, and twist it to your right side by bringing the left hand to the right side at shoulder height.
- Return to the starting position, and then repeat on the other side.
- Perform it for the mentioned reps, alternating the reps between the sides.

Note:

If your core is not strong enough, you might need to use the hand on the floor for further assistance. By pushing on the floor, it helps make performing the sit-up easier. Overtime, you`ll do it without assistance, as shown in the image.

BRUSHING BODY DOWN

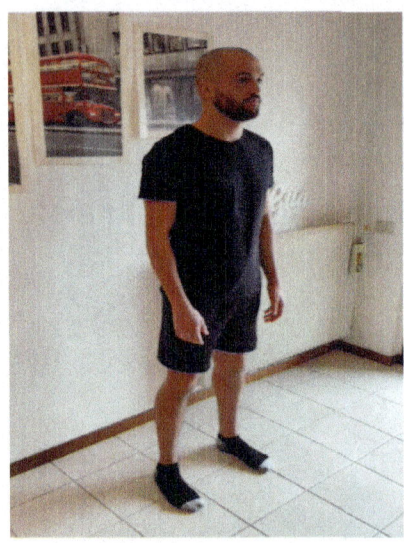

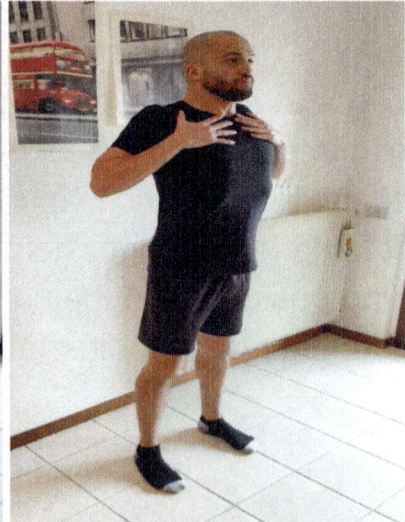

Step 1 - Stand up and relax your body.

Step 2 - Bring your hands to your chest.

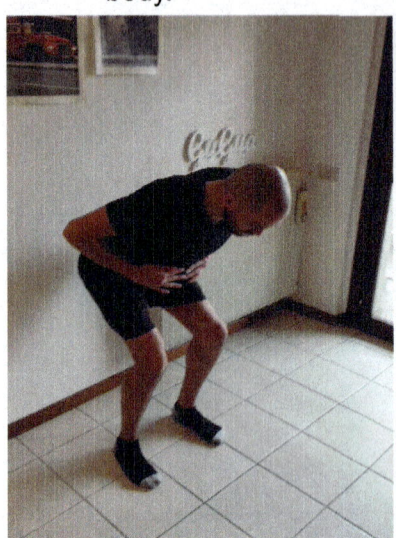

Step 3 - Brush them down towards your belly.

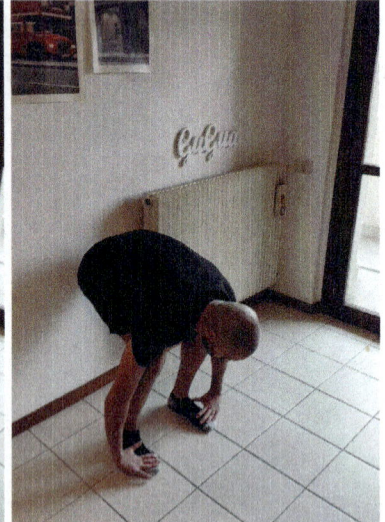

Step 4 - Then, reach your feet.

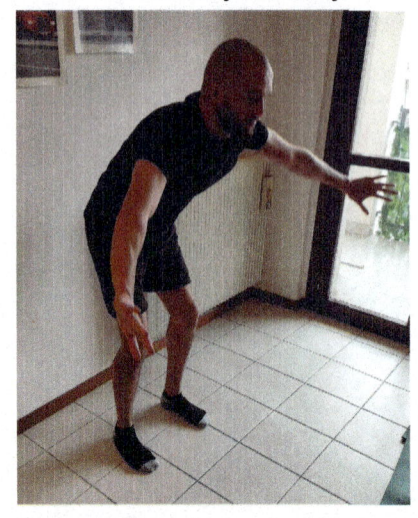

Step 5 - Push inner tension away with your hands exhaling fully. Then, repeat from Step 1.

How to do it:

- Step 1: Stand with feet shoulder-width apart and arms next to the body.
- Step 2: Bring your hands to chest height as if you want to start brushing away your bad feelings and stress from there.
- Step 3: Imagine brushing it down your body and reaching pelvic height.
- Step 4: Keep going down, reaching your feet. Bend your knees, not just your back.
- Step 5: Lastly, push the feelings away and outside. Exhale fully from your mouth as you do so.
- Come back to the starting position and repeat for the mentioned number of times.

Note:

To fully experience the benefits of the exercise, vividly imagine brushing away the stress and anxiety you feel in your chest outside of the body. Exhale deeply while performing the movement, and inhale when returning to the starting positlon.

OPEN HEART

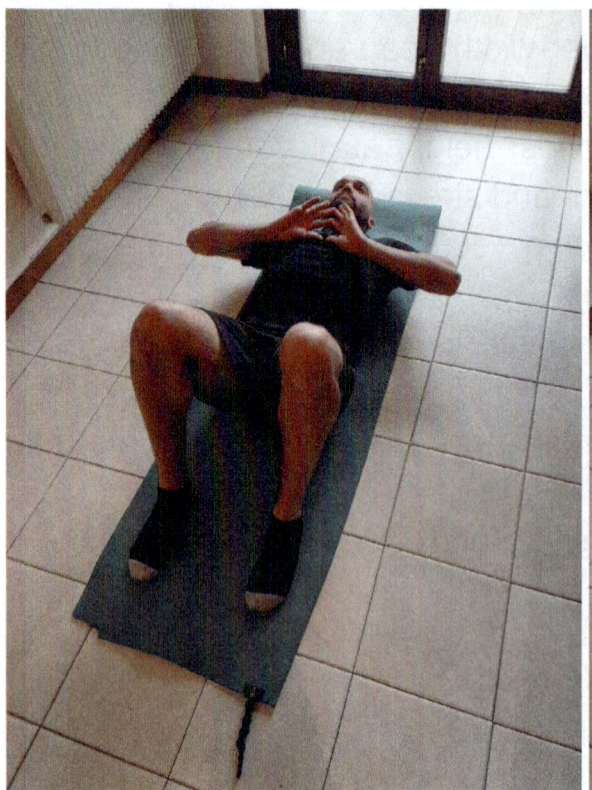

Step 1 - Lie on the mat with knees bent and feet on the floor, hands at chest height fingers in contact, elbows wide.

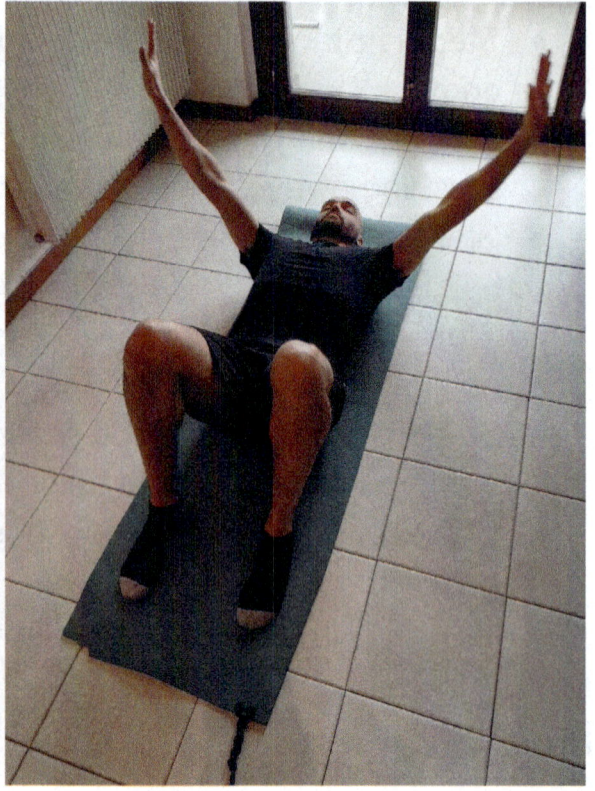

Step 2 - Imagine pushing something out of your chest in front of you. Extend your arms as you do so.

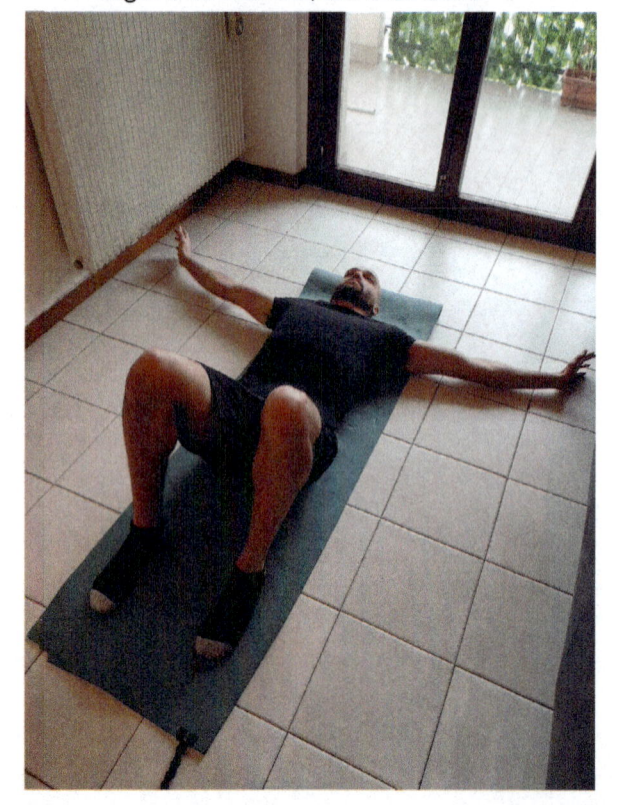

Step 3 - Bring the hands wide, releasing all the tension accumulated. Lastly, come back to the starting position, and repeat for the mentioned reps.

How to do it:

- Lie on the mat with knees bent and feet on the floor, hands at chest height, elbows wide, as in Step 1. Find your center and peace.
- Exhale via your nose, and imagine throwing something out of your chest in front of you, then slowly widen your arms as in Step 2.
- Bring the hands wide and onto the floor as in Step 3.
- Lastly, inhale and come back to the starting position. Repeat it for the mentioned number of times.

Note:

Focus on the feelings you have during the exercise. Use the first step to find your center and imagine throwing outside your body the anxiety stored in your chest area. Exhale deeply while performing the exercise.

KNEE GRAB LYING

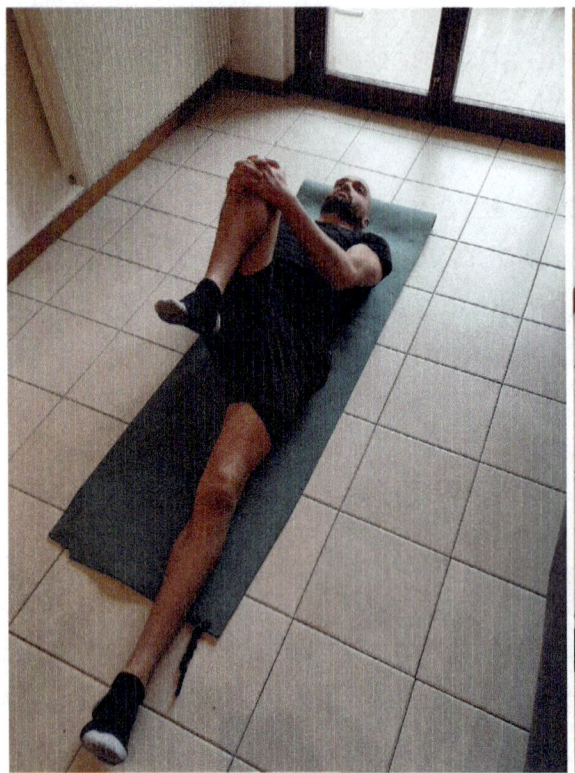

Step 1 - Lie on your back with the left leg extended and the right knee close to the chest, hugged by your hands.

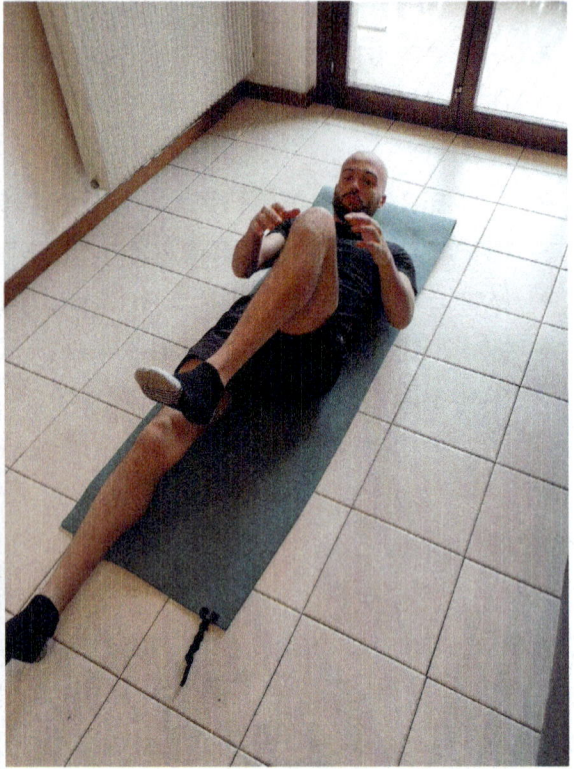

Step 2 - Then, bring the right leg down and bring the left one up close to the chest.

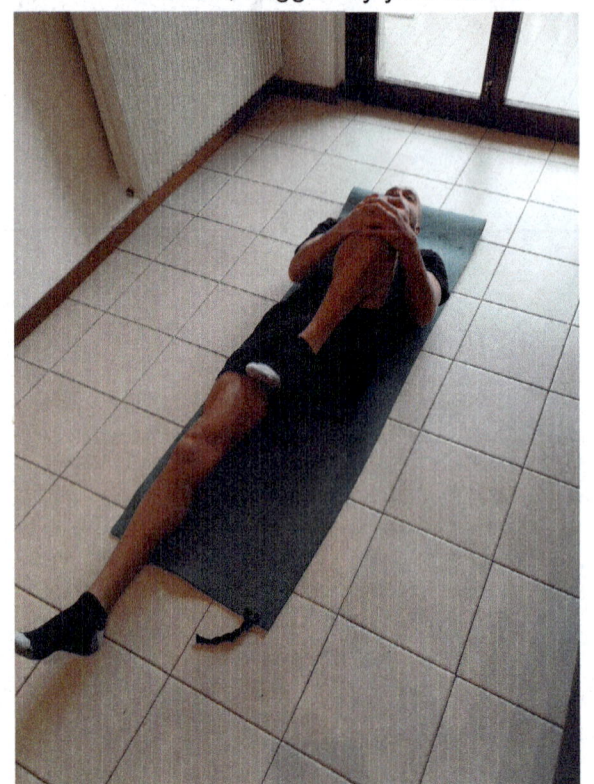

Step 3 - Hold this position for 3 seconds, and then repeat on the other side.

How to do it:

- Lie on your back with the left leg extended and the right knee in contact with your chest, hugged by your hands. Relax your shoulders and neck on the mat, relaxed. Exhale while bringing the knee to your chest. Keep the back aligned on the mat. Maintain the position for 3 seconds.
- Switch legs. Bring the right one down first, and then bring the left one up. Perform the movement slowly and controlled.
- Repeat it on the other side, holding the position for 3 seconds - exhale fully.
- Perform the movement for the mentioned number of times, alternating the sides.

Note:

Perform the movement slowly for maximum benefits. Remember to exhale through your mouth. This is a great exercise to improve flexibility. If you struggle with bringing the knee close to the chest while keeping the back on the mat, don't worry. Focus on keeping the back on the mat and bring the knee as close as possible to the chest. You will get better the more your practice.

KNEE GRAB SEATED

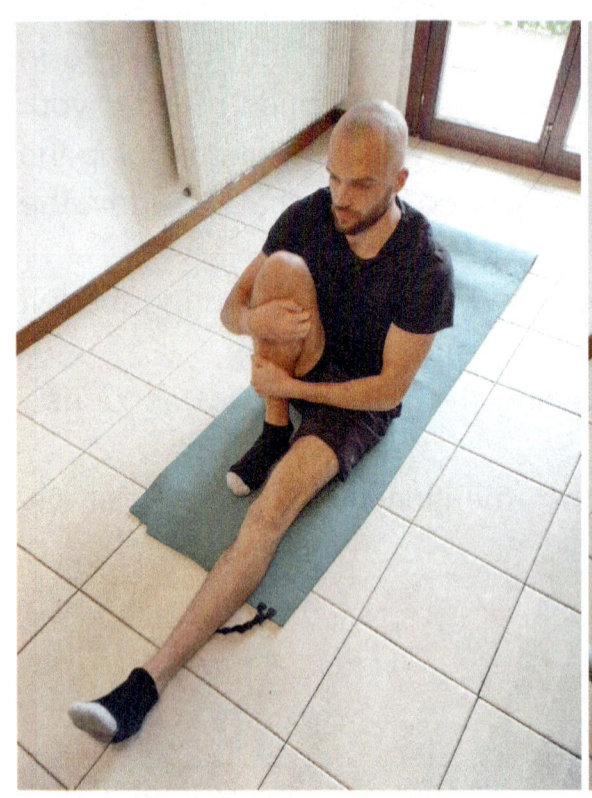

Step 1 - Sit on the mat with a straight back, left leg extended, and right leg hugged by your hands against the chest.

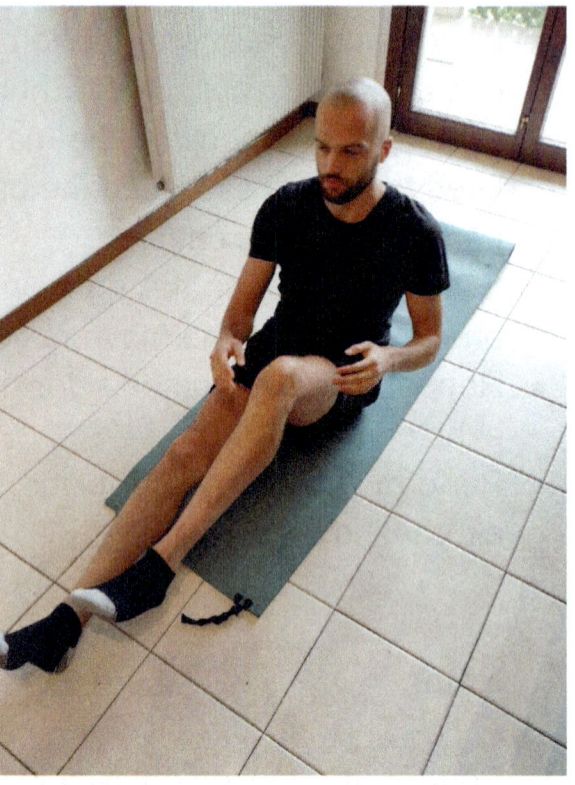

Step 2 - Switch legs. Bring the right one down first and then bring the left one up.

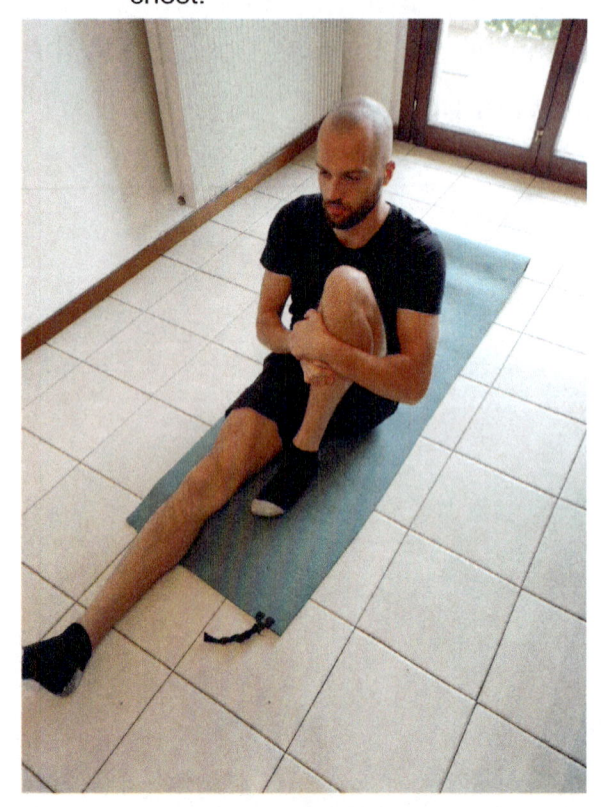

Step 3 - Repeat it on the other side.

How to do it:

- Sit on the mat with a straight back, left leg extended, and right leg hugged by your hands against the chest. Hold the position for 3 seconds, trying to gently squeeze the leg against your chest, feeling the tension in your legs dissipate as you squeeze them against your chest
- Switch legs. Bring the right one down first and then bring the left one up. Perform this very gently, holding it for 3 seconds
- Perform it for the mentioned number of times, alternating the sides.

Note:

To maximize your flexibility, perform this movement slowly and exhale through your mouth. If you have difficulty bringing the knee close to your chest while keeping your back straight, don't worry. It will get easier if you focus on keeping your back straight and bringing the knee as close to your chest as possible.

GROIN RELEASE

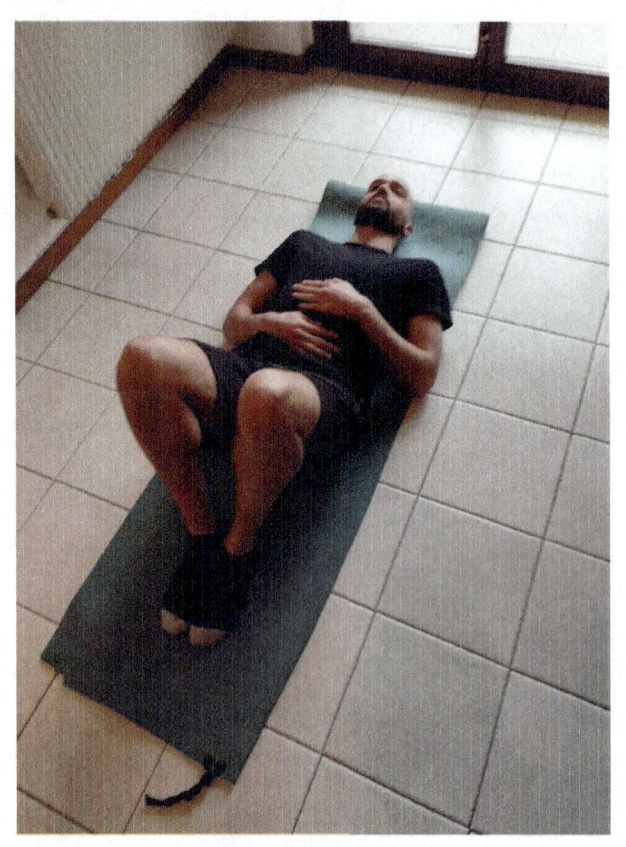

Step 1 - Lie on your back with your hands on your belly, knees bent, and feet on the floor.

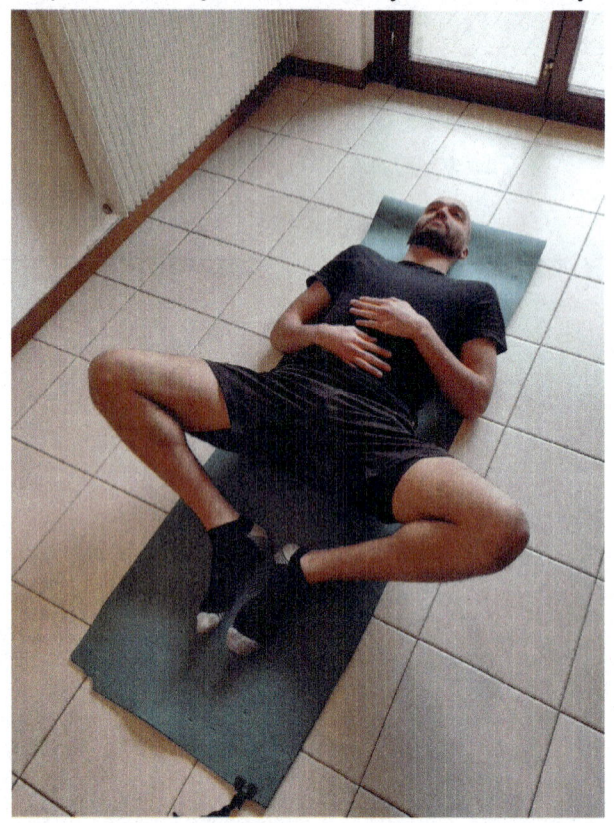

Step 2 - Exhale and gently widen your knees. Then, come back to the starting position and repeat the movement for the mentioned reps.

How to do it:

- Lie on your back with your hands on your belly, knees bent, and feet on the floor. Once you are in this position, take a few deep breaths before starting to get rid of excessive tension you might have in some parts of your body.
- Then, exhale from your mouth and gently widen your knees. Bring your soles together and widen your groins as much as possible. Keep the position for 5 seconds, relaxing fully into it.
- Then slowly come back to the starting position. Repeat the movement for the mentioned reps.

Note:

Keep your lower back on the floor while doing the exercise by breathing deeply while doing it. The hip/groin area is usually stiff because of a sedentary lifestyle. This exercise will help loosen up the muscles and tension that has built up. It is a great exercise for groin health and to let go of anxiety.

SOMATIC HIP MOVEMENT

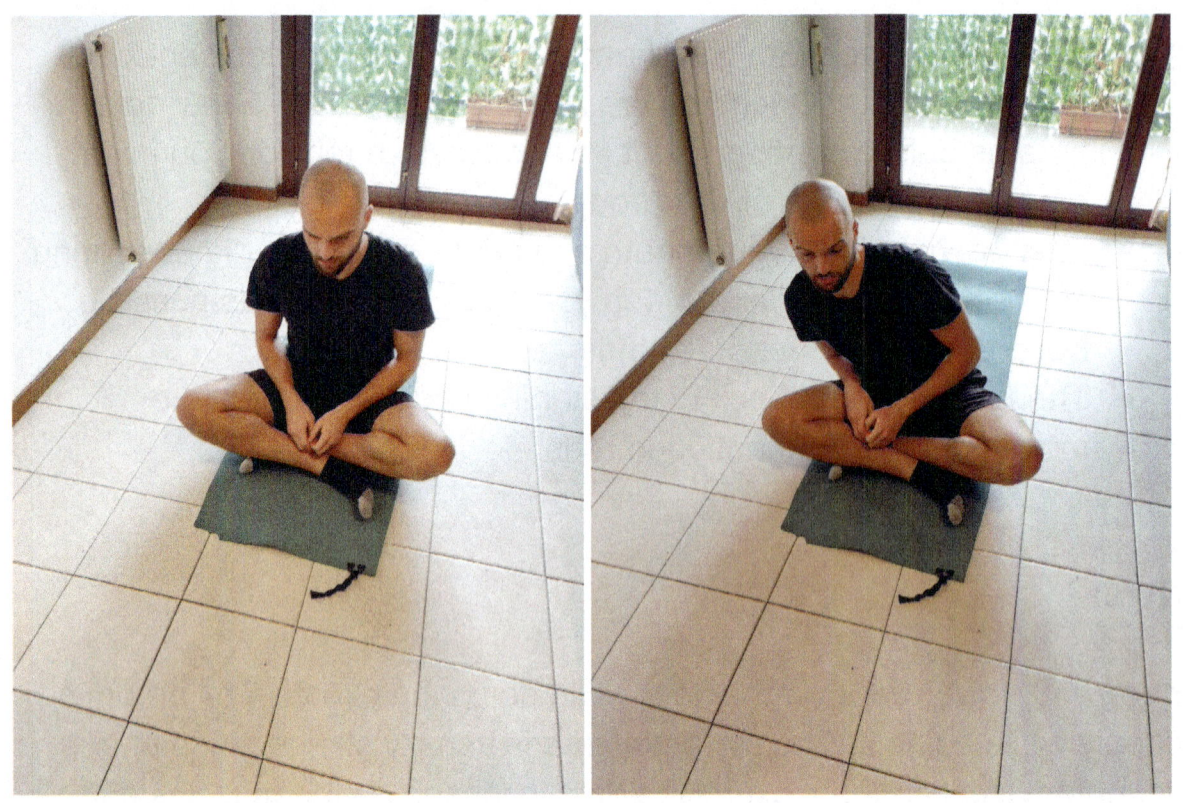

Step 1 - Sit on the mat with legs crossed and an erect spine. Breathe gently.

Step 2 - Shift your torso and body weight to the right. Hold the position for 1 second,

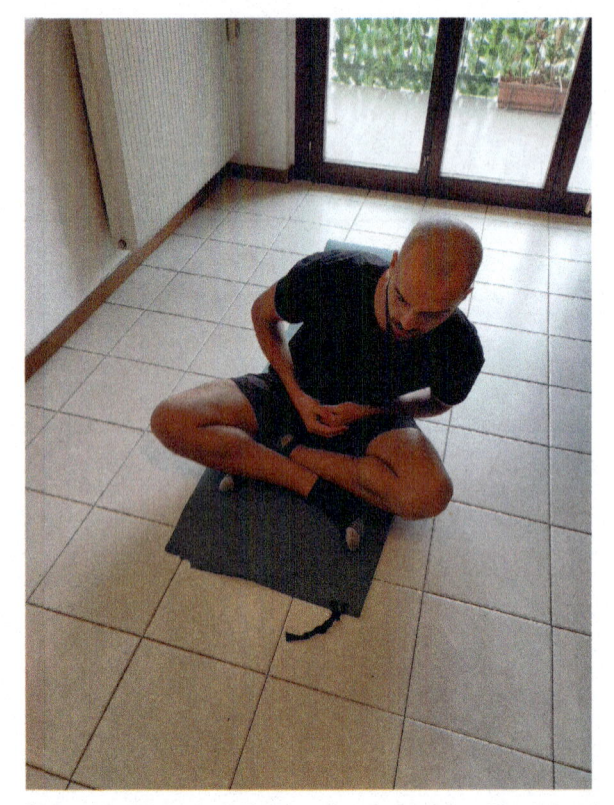

Step 3 - Then, shift it to the left side. Repeat the sequence from Step 1 for the mentioned seconds.

How to do it:

- Sit on the mat with legs crossed and an erect spine. Hands can be kept on your lap. Exhale fully first. Then, keep breathing gently through your nose.
- Shift your torso and body weight to the right side. Hold the position for 1 second.
- From there, start shifting your body weight towards the left side, as shown in Step 3.
- Repeat the sequence for the mentioned seconds.

Note:

Find a rhythm and try to move your body as fluidly as possible. It is an exercise done for your hips and to develop a mind-body connection.

PUSH OUT IN FRONT

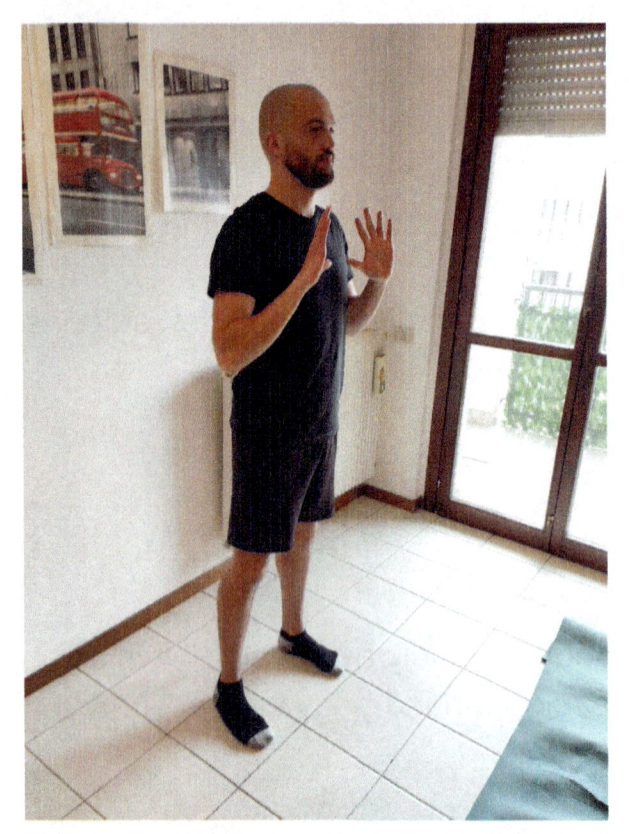

Step 1 - Stand with hands at chest height. Look in front of you. Inhale as you are in this position.

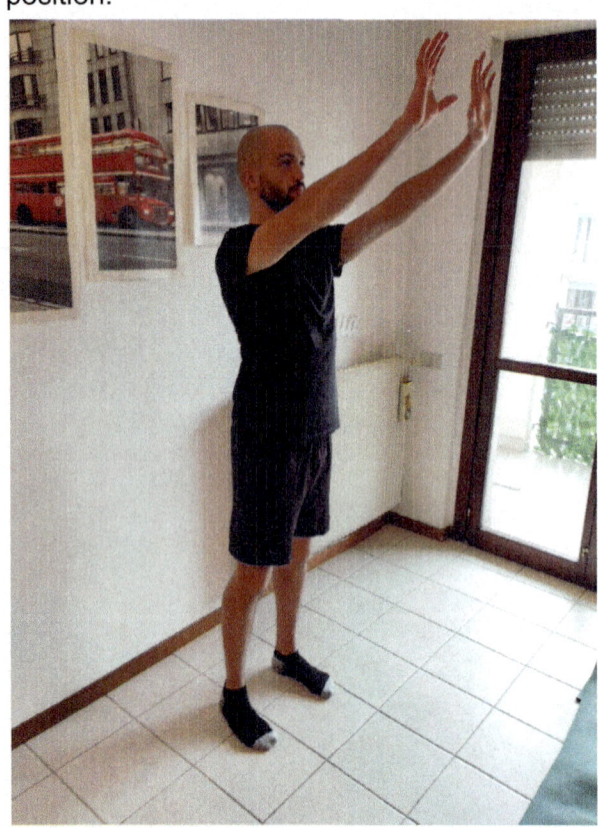

Step 2 - Push your arms forward and upward without lifting your eyes. Exhale as you perform the movement, imagining to get rid of all negative energy inside you.

How to do it:

- Stand with your hands at chest height. Keep the hands there as if you are holding a ball that you have to throw. Take a deep inhale through your nose.
- Exhale, and focus on getting rid of all the negative energy inside you, and push your arms forward and upward as if you are throwing the ball.
- Come back to the starting position, and perform it for the mentioned reps.

Note:

This helps to "push out" traumas. Inhale while bringing the hands back, and exhale while pushing out. The pushing out movement should be done quickly, while the comeback to the starting position should be done more slowly. Imagine you are throwing stress and trauma away from your body.

SKIING

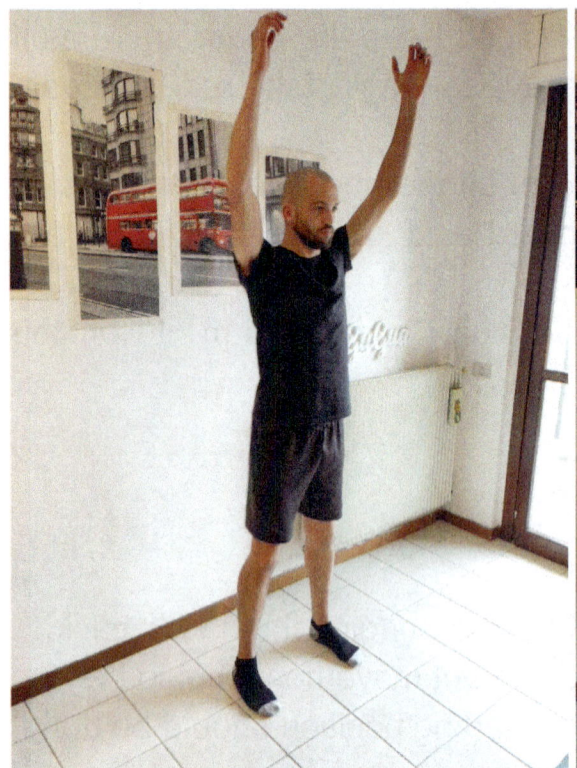

Step 1 - Stand with feet slightly wider than shoulder-width apart, arms extended above your head.

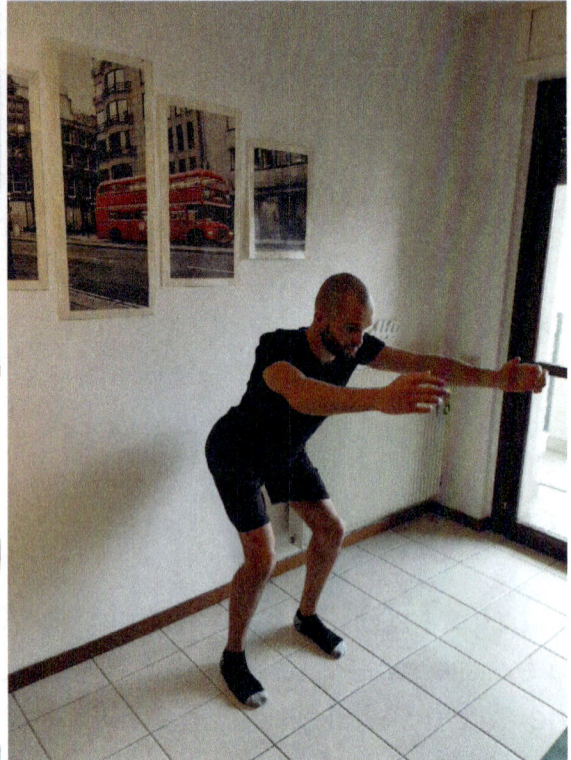

Step 2 - Swing your arms down and bend your knees, bringing your butt back.. Keep your arms straight.

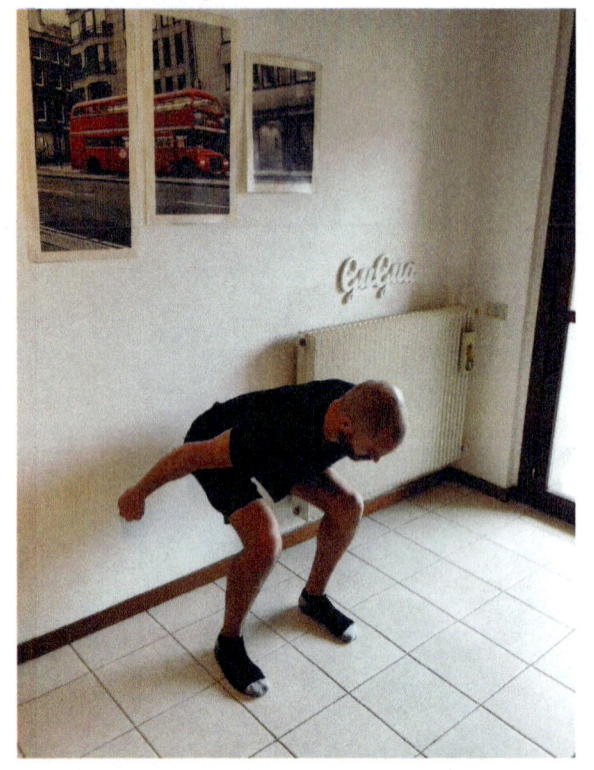

Step 3 - Swing your arms backward and bend your knees close to 90 degrees, bringing your chest close to your thighs. Repeat the sequence for the mentioned seconds.

How to do it:

- Stand with feet slightly wider than shoulder-width apart, arms extended above your head as in Step 1.
- Swing the hands down and bend your knees, bringing your butt back as in Step 2.
- Swing hands backward and bend your knees close to 90 degrees, bringing your chest close to your thighs, imagining to be a skier as in Step 3.
- Come back to the starting position, and repeat it for the mentioned seconds.

Note:

The main focus here is imagining you have all the tension and anxiety in your hands, and as you perform the movement you get rid of it by pushing it back. Exhale while performing the movement and inhale when coming back to the starting position.

Also, this is a great physical exercise; the faster it is performed, the harder it is - Alternating more gentle exercises to more intense ones is great to get rid of toxins in your body as well as release bad thoughts and emotional trauma.

SOMATIC SHAKING

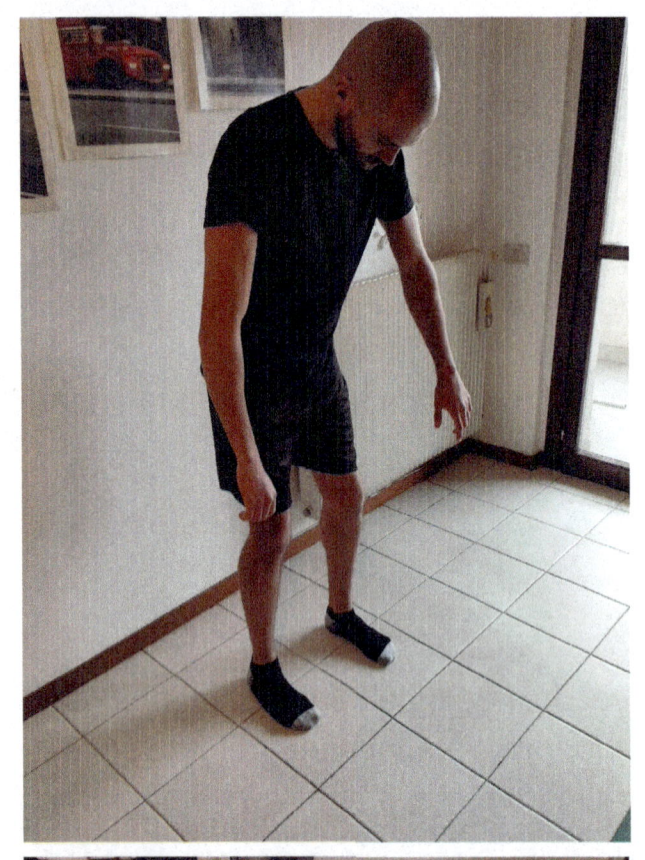

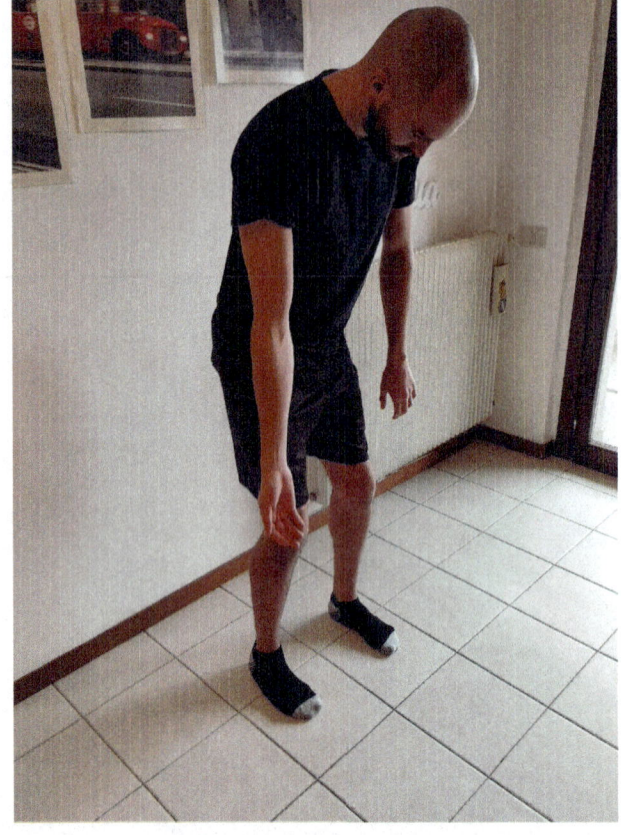

The act of shaking tension and trauma from your body is shown in both pictures by moving without a pattern. It is a full-body shake.

How to do it:

- This exercise is a full-body shake called 'Somatic Shaking.' It is designed to release tension, anxiety, unhappiness, and stress from your body. Remember to use every part of your body, from your feet to your head; the whole body has to move and shake off the bad energy.
- Repeat it for the mentioned seconds.

Note:

It is crucial to focus on the negative energy and feelings within yourself in order to eliminate them. This will help you get the best out of this exercise and feel better just after 60 seconds!.

HIP ROCKING ON STOMACH

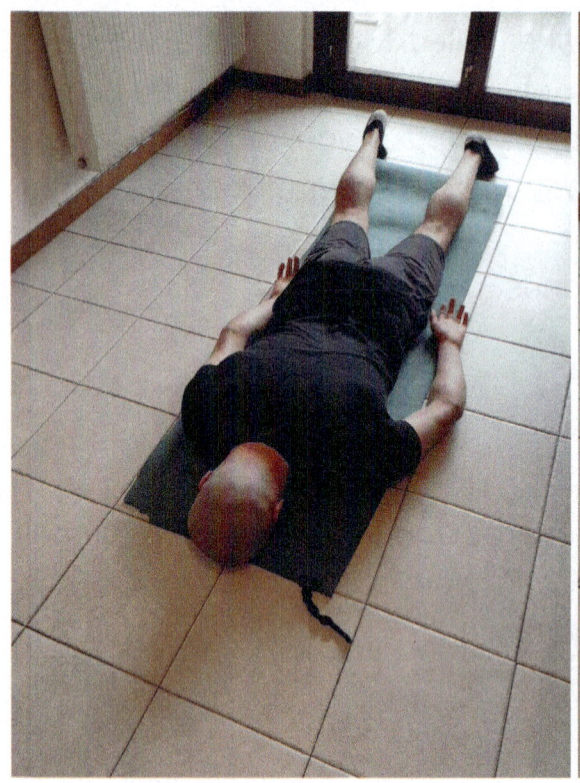

Step 1 - Lie on the floor facing down, arms next to the body.

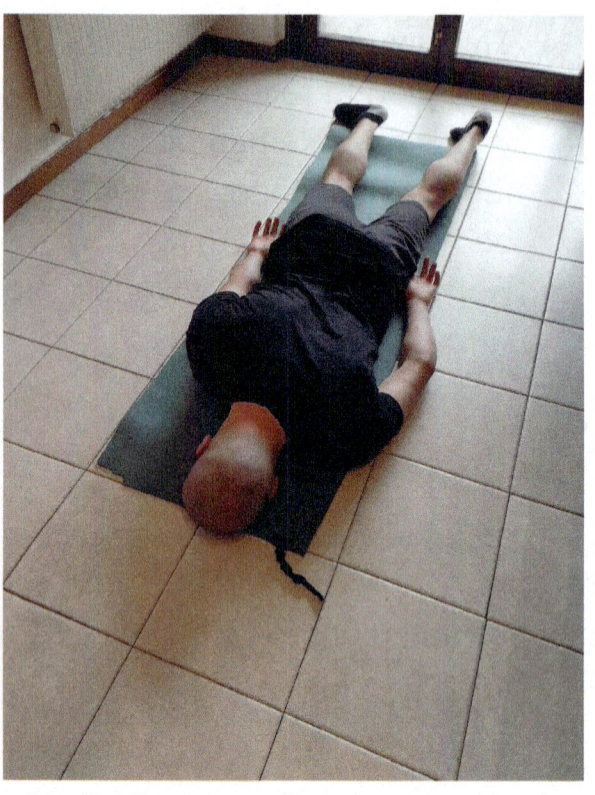

Step 2 - Rock your whole body from side to Side. Starting from the left side.

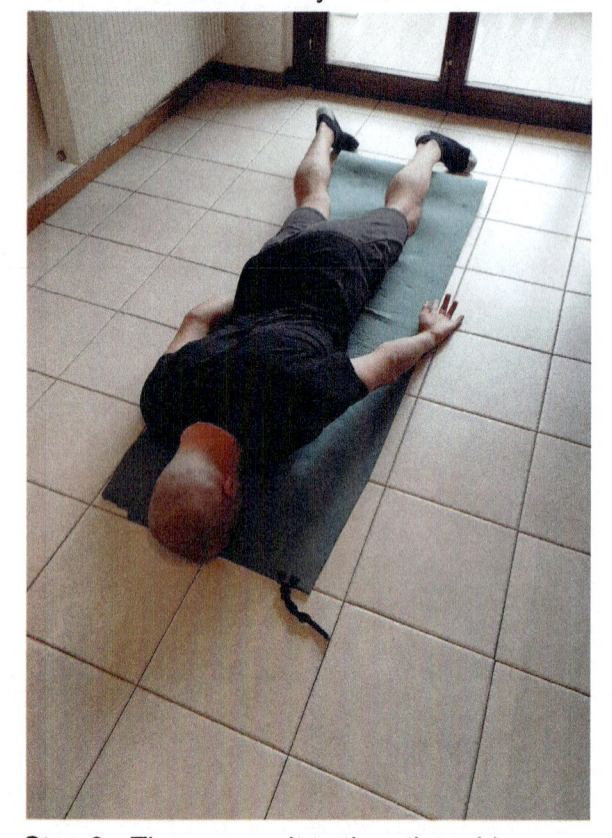

Step 3 - Then, move it to the other side.

How to do it:

- Lie on the floor facing down, with your arms next to your body. Relax all your muscles.
- Gently rock your body left and right, feeling your body weight shifting, paying attention to your body's sensations.
- Perform the exercise for the mentioned duration of seconds.

Note:

This exercise is great for releasing trauma; just let it go and keep rocking. It should feel nice.

LATERAL LUNGE AND REACH

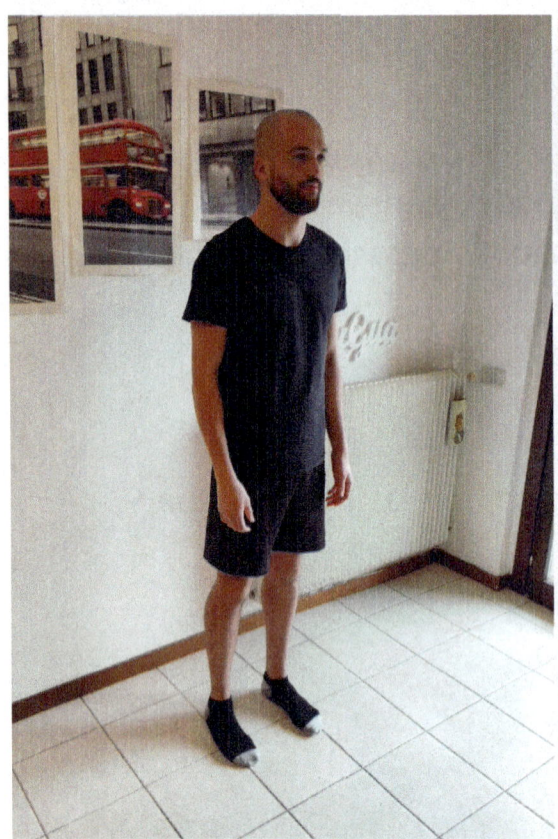

Step 1 - Stand straight with arms next to your body.

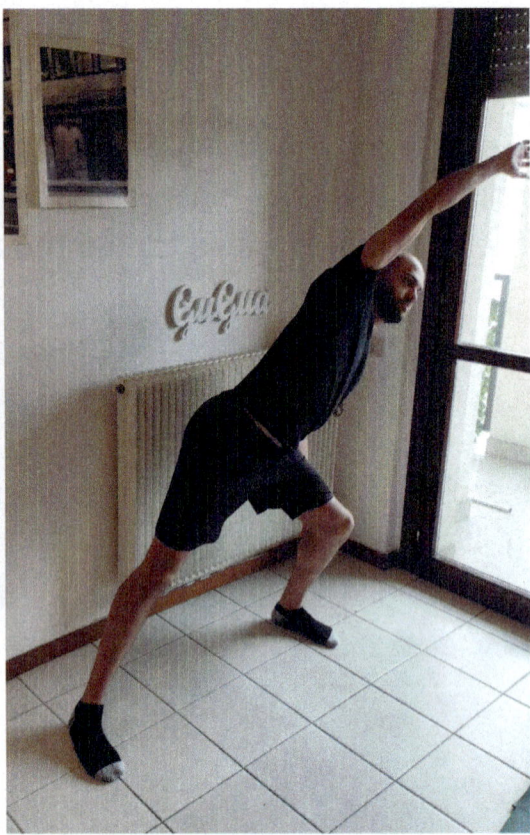

Step 2 - Step with the left foot to the side, bending your left knee while reaching with your right hand over your left side.

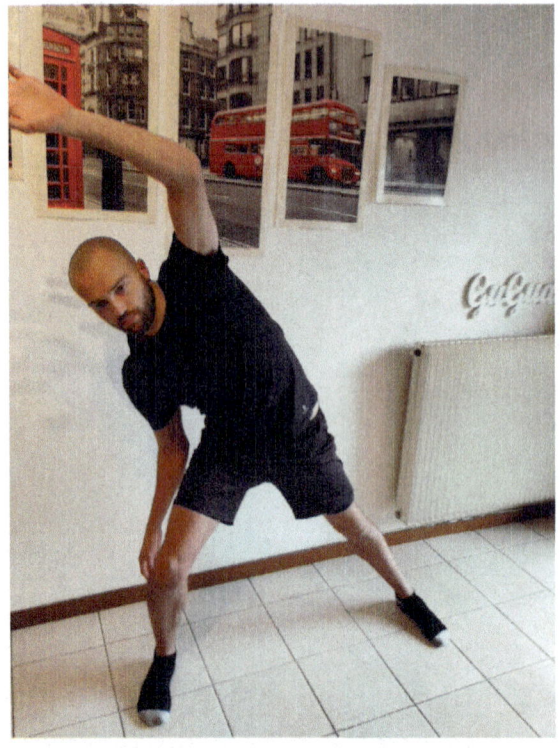

Step 3 - Then, come back to the starting position, and perform it on the other side.

How to do it:

- Stand with arms next to your body. Exhale gently before starting to move
- Step your left foot towards the left side, and bend your left knee as you do so, keeping your right leg straight.
- Reach with your right hand over your left side. You should feel a burning sensation in your left quad and glute as well as a stretch on the right side of your back. Reach over with your right hand as high and as wide as possible, leaning your body towards the left. Hold the position for 2 seconds, exhaling fully.
- Then, slowly come back to the starting position - inhale as you do so - and repeat it on the other side, performing the movement for the mentioned reps, alternating the sides.

Note:

Control your breathing, perform the exercise slowly, and focus on the muscles involved and on your feelings.

FAWN

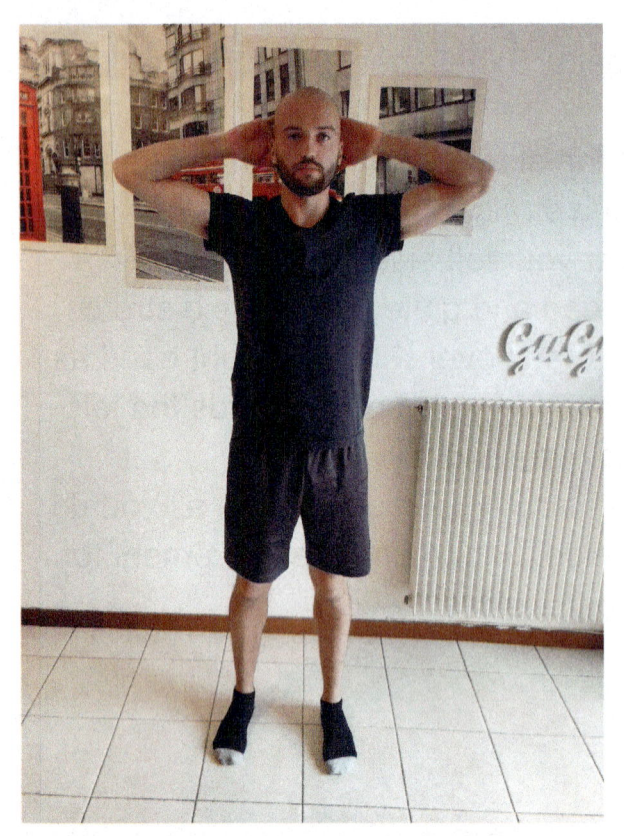

Step 1 - Stand with feet shoulder-width apart and hands behind your head.

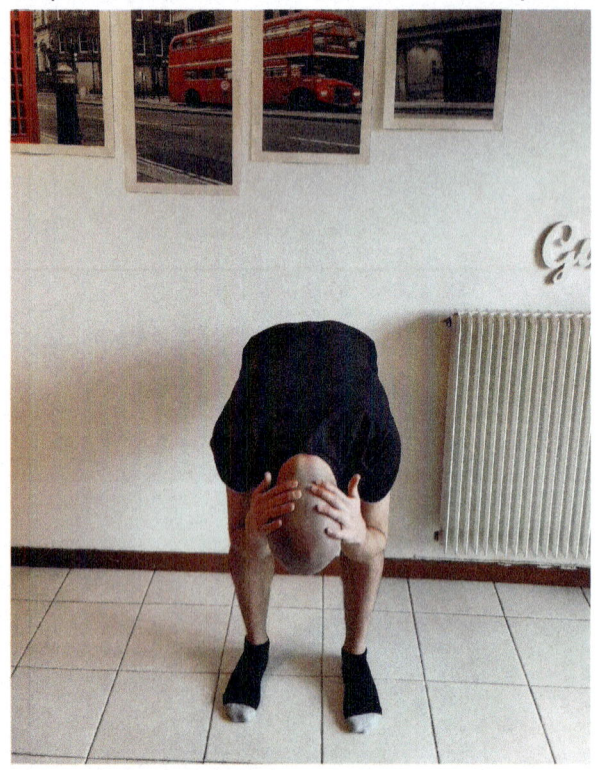

Step 2 - Exhale deeply through your mouth while rounding your spine and bringing elbows against knees. Inhale as you come back to the starting position. Repeat for the mentioned reps.

How to do it:

- Stand with feet shoulder-width apart and hands behind your head, as shown in Step 1. Inhale deeply while in this position.
- Then, exhale deeply while rounding your spine and bringing elbows against knees as shown in Step 2. Let go of tensions, anxiety, and trauma. Focus on relaxing the muscle of your posterior chain (glutes, back, neck and back of the thighs).
- Inhale and come back to the starting position. Repeat for the mentioned number of times.

Note:

Focus on your feelings and sensations while performing the exercise. To maximize the benefits, imagine exhaling your stress, anxiety, and all the negative feelings you might store in your body.

DOWNWARD DOG

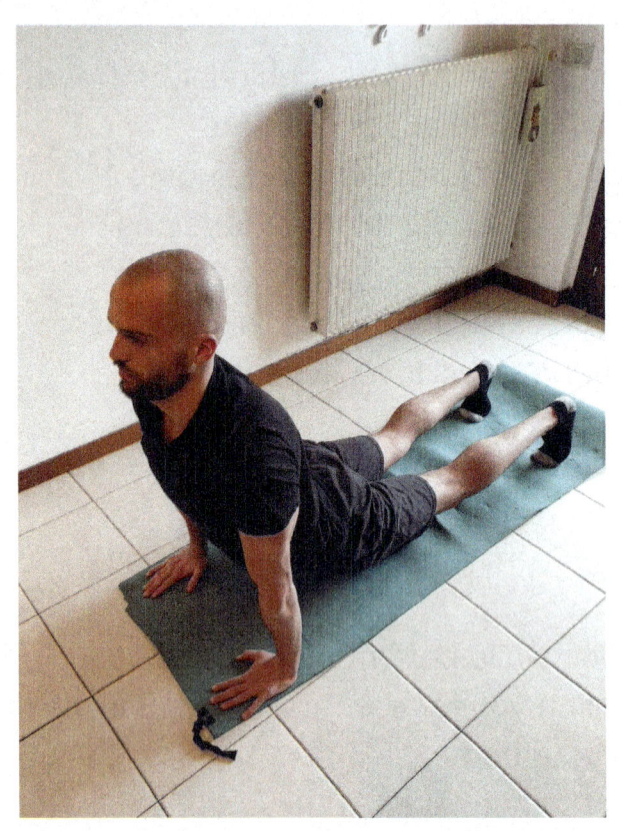

Step 1 - Start on the mat with feet and hands on the floor. Keep your entire body elevated and keep your chest up and arms straight.

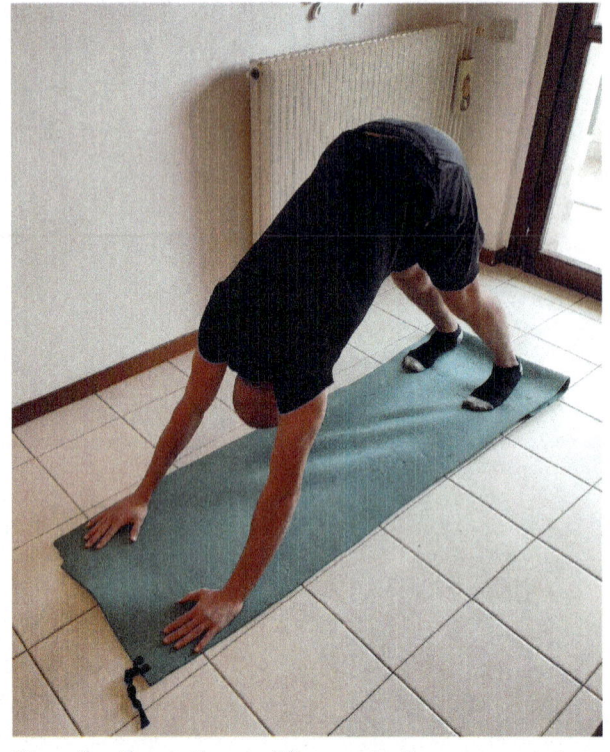

Step 2 - From there, lift your butt up as much as possible while keeping your feet and hands on the mat. Hold the position for 1 second, and then come back into the starting position.

How to do it:

- Start on the mat with feet and hands on the floor. Keep your entire body elevated, arms straight and chest up.
  This position requires strength and flexibility. Inhale while in this position.
- Then, exhale as you lift your butt up as much as possible while keeping your feet and hands on the mat, as shown in Step 2. Ensure your legs and back are straight, as if you are trying to create a triangle with the mat being the other side. Hold the position for 1 second.
- Come back to the starting position, and repeat it for the specified number of times.

Note:

Focus on breathing and concentrate on stretching and relaxing only the muscles that you need. Do not tense your body. This exercise is great to stretch your posterior chain that tends to be stiff for most people due to a sedentary lifestyle.

If you feel too much stretch on the back of your leg as you lift the hips up - Step 2 - feel free to slightly bend your knees. Over time you'll be able to do the exercise without bending them.

ROBOT

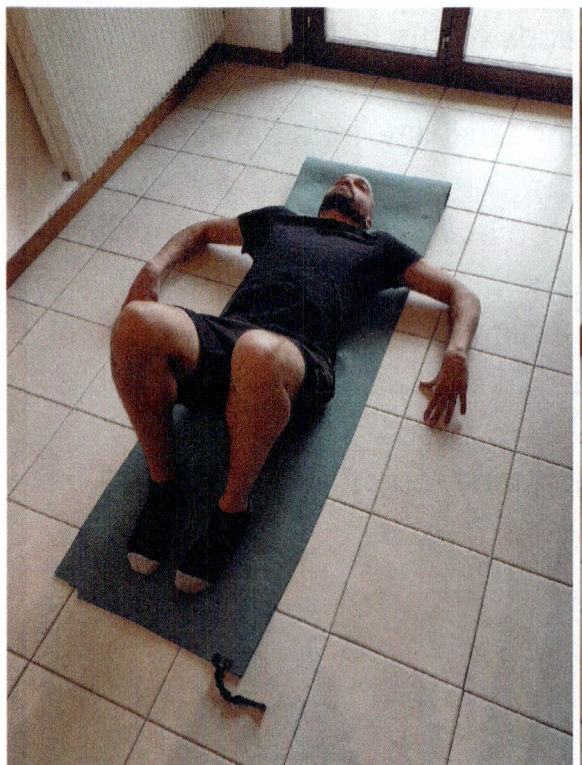

Step 1 - Lie on your back, knees bent and feet on the floor. Arms wide, elbows bent 90 degrees.

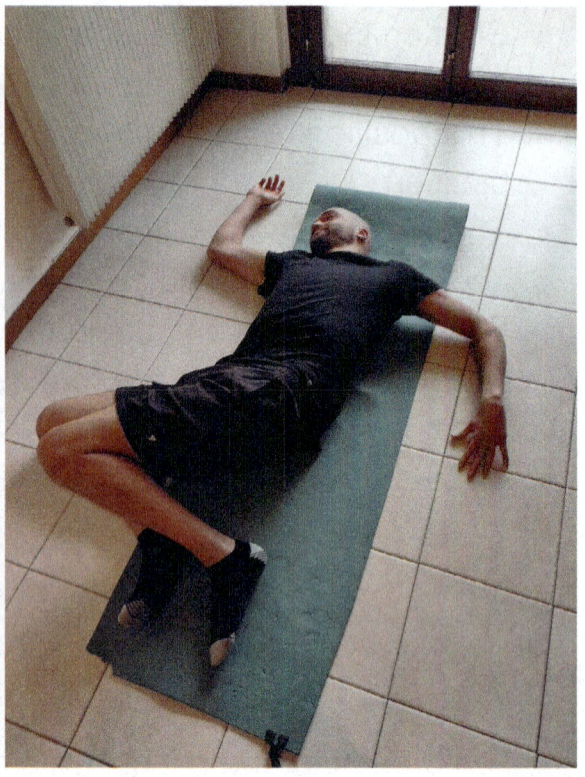

Step 2 - Rotate right elbow up. Turn your face towards the right and rotate hips right by falling the right knees on the mat.

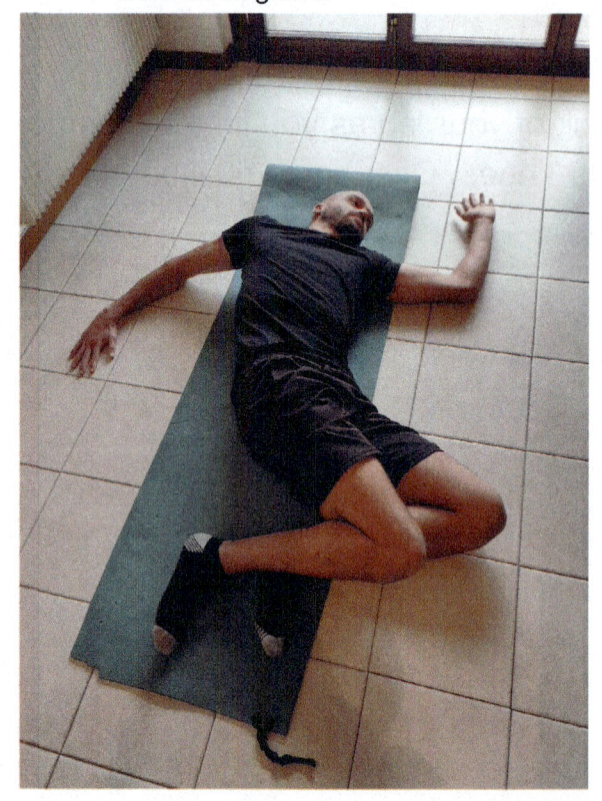

Step 3 - Then, repeat it on the other side. Perform the reps as mentioned in the plan.

How to do it:

- Lie on your back with knees bent and feet on the floor. Keep your arms wide, elbows bent at 90 degrees. Relax your neck and avoid tensing your muscles.
- Rotate your right elbow up, turn your face towards the right, and rotate your hips to the right by lowering the right knee to the mat.
- Repeat on the other side, and keep performing the movement for the mentioned seconds.

Note:

Keep breathing gently without holding your body. This will help to avoid tensing your body while performing the movement. Ideally it should be smooth and fluid movement.

PIGEON POSE

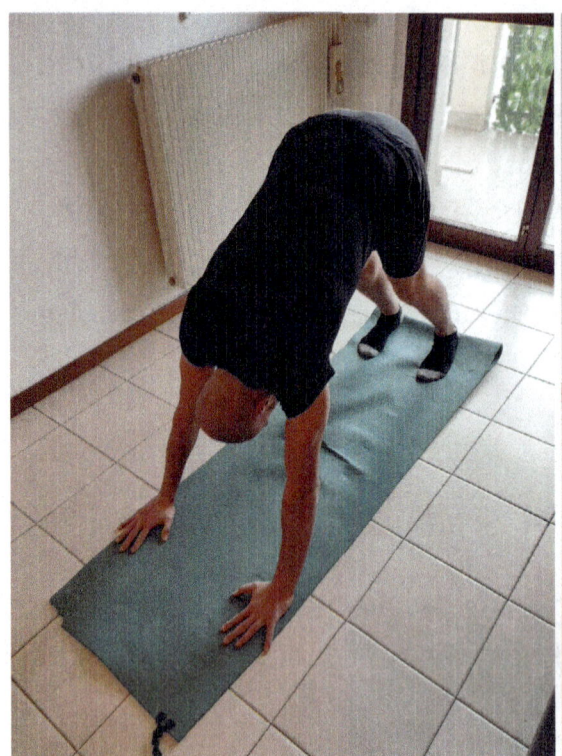

Step 1 - Start with feet and hands on the, mat. Lift your butt as much as you can.

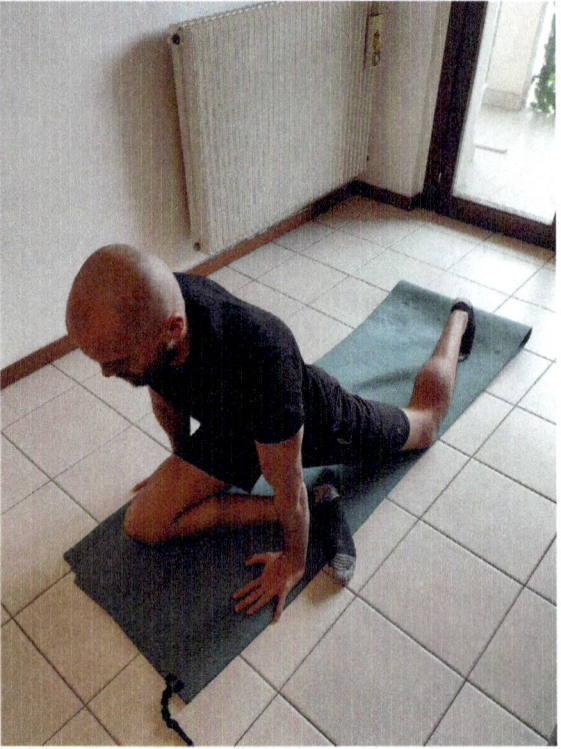

Step 2 - Bring the right knee to the floor and place the right ankle between your left leg and your left arm.

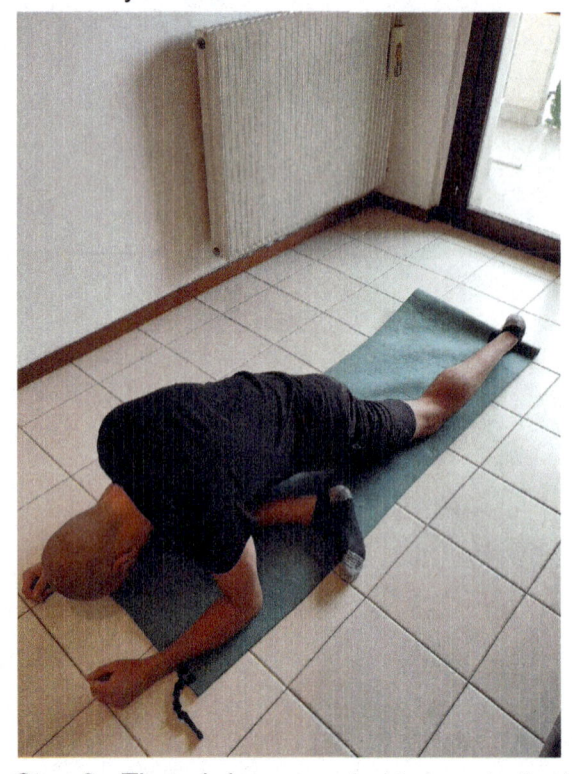

Step 3 - Then, bring your chest close to the knee as much as you can, and the lateral side of Use your elbows for balance. Then, come back into the starting position and repeat on the other side.

How to do it:

- Start with feet and hands on the mat, straight spine, and legs. Lift your butt as much as possible. Keep your back straight. You should feel a gentle stretch on your calves as you get into this position.
- From there, bring the right knee to the floor as shown, and the right ankle between your left leg and left arm. Perform the movement slowly. You should feel a stretch in your right glute as you get into this position,
- Exhale fully, and bring your chest close to the knee - use arms for assistance if needed - and the lateral side of the thigh should be in touch with the mat. Hold the position for one full breath.
- Come back to the starting position and repeat on the other side.
- Repeat it for the mentioned number of times, alternating the sides.

Note:

If step 3 looks too difficult, simply do your best to bring your chest close to the floor. If you cannot do it, no problem. With practice you'll improve your hip flexibility, and your movement will be more fluid,a s you get rid of unnecessary tension.

BREATHING CIRCLE

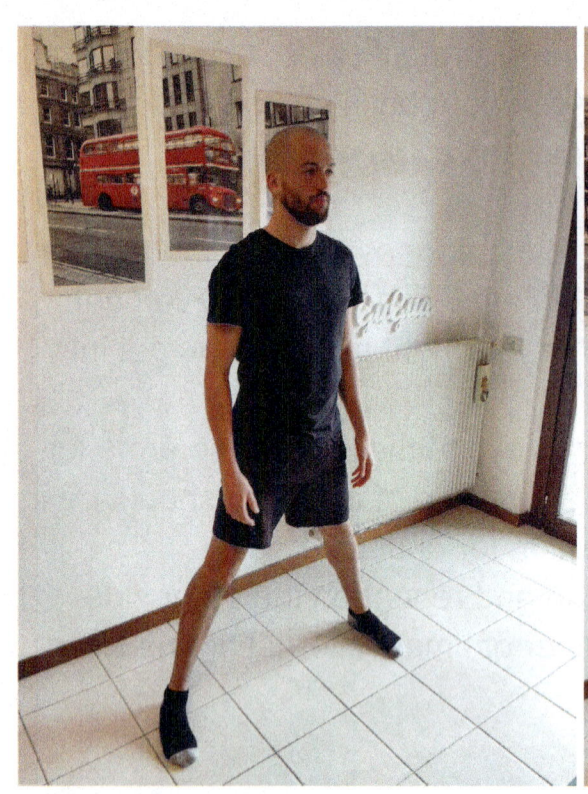

Step 1 - Start standing and spread your legs.

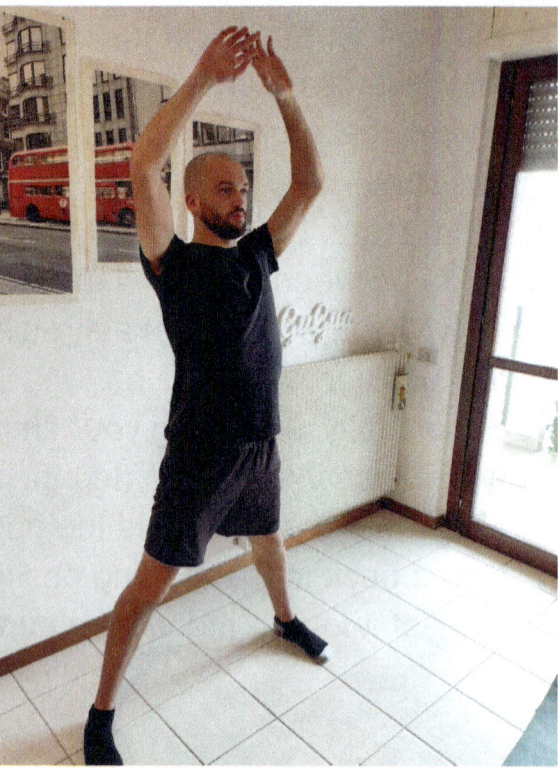

Step 2 - Bring your arms over your head and inhale deeply as you do so.

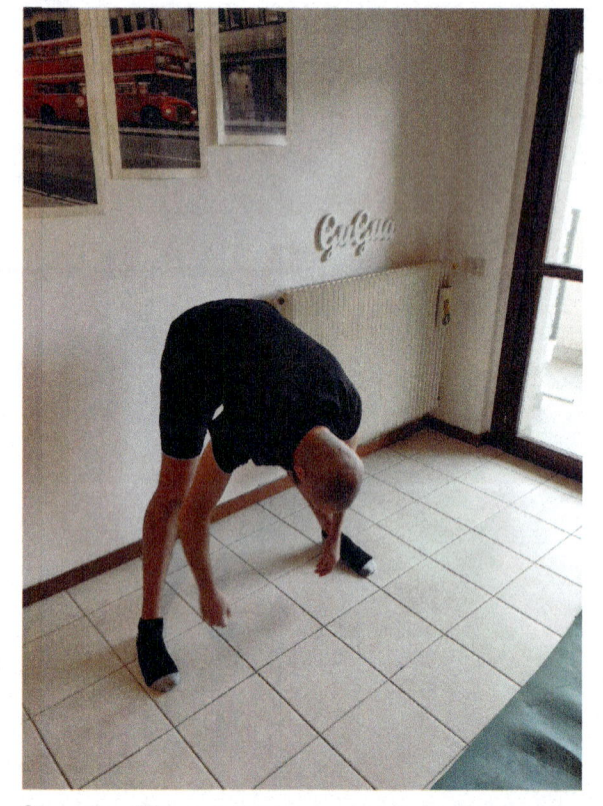

Step 3 - Then, bring your trunk and arms down towards the floor exhaling fully, releasing all your emotions. Then, come back to step 1 and repeat.

How to do it:

- Stand and spread your legs while having your arms to the side. Exhale fully before starting.
- Bring your arms over your head and inhale through your nose fully inflating your chest - This step will last one to two seconds.
- Then, bring your trunk and arms down towards the floor exhaling fully, releasing all your emotions, as shown in step 3 - This step will last two to three seconds, slightly longer than step 1.
- Then, come back to the starting position and repeat for the mentioned reps.

Note:

Great exercise to get in touch with your body and find relief in just a few deep breaths. The more you can spread your leg the better it is, especially as you exhale and release your back.

PUSH WALL

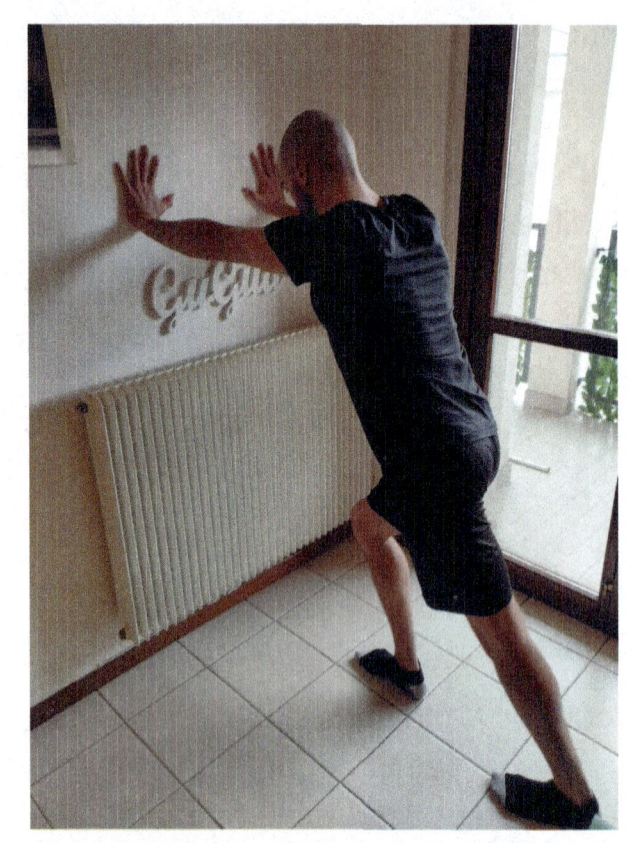

Step 1 - Push the wall for 5 seconds with all the force you have.

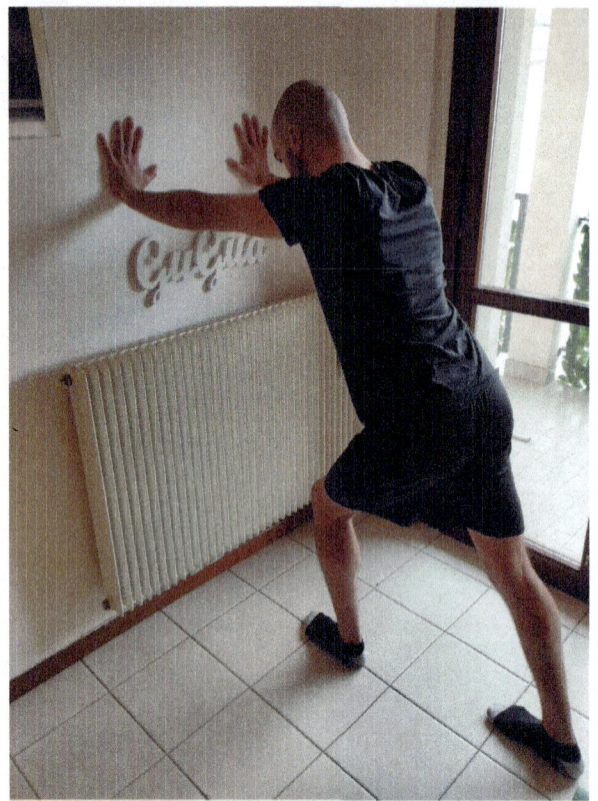

Step 2 - Then, take a few seconds rest, and repeat switching legs. Keep alternating the reps as mentioned in the plan.

How to do it:

- Start standing a few feet from the wall. Push it with your hands for 5 seconds with all the force you have. Focus on "pushing" the stress and anxiety away as you do so.
- Release for a few seconds, and do it on the other side.
- Keep alternating the movement for the mentioned reps.

Note:

Discharge energy to allow the body to release anger by pushing something. It also strengthens your arms.

STOMP YOUR HEELS

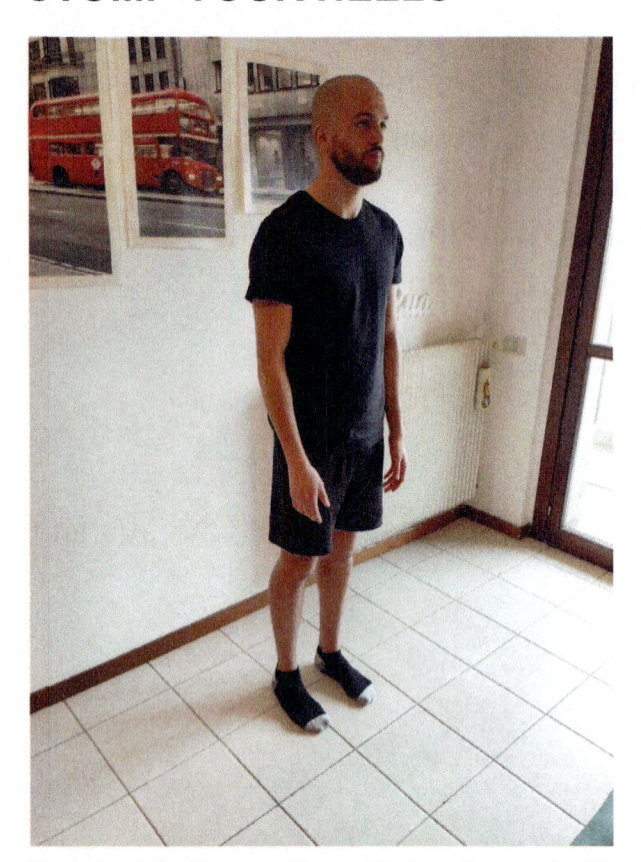

Step 1 - Starting position with feet flat on the floor.

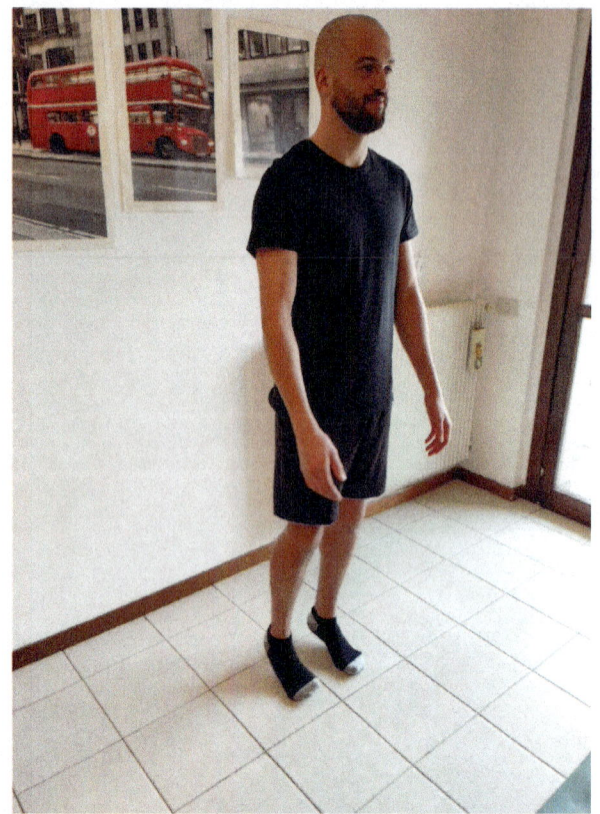

Step 2 - Lift your heels slightly. Then quickly come back to the starting position. Keep stomping your heels for the mentioned seconds.

How to do it:

- Start by standing with feet flat on the floor and arms at your sides.
- Lift your heels slightly, then return to the starting position as quickly as possible.
- Continue stomping your heels for the mentioned duration in seconds. The quicker the better.

Note:

Doing the exercise might seem easy. However, if you consistently stomp your heels for the specified duration while keeping your entire body relaxed, you will notice some shaking. This is excellent for releasing tension and letting go in the present moment.

RUN SHAKE

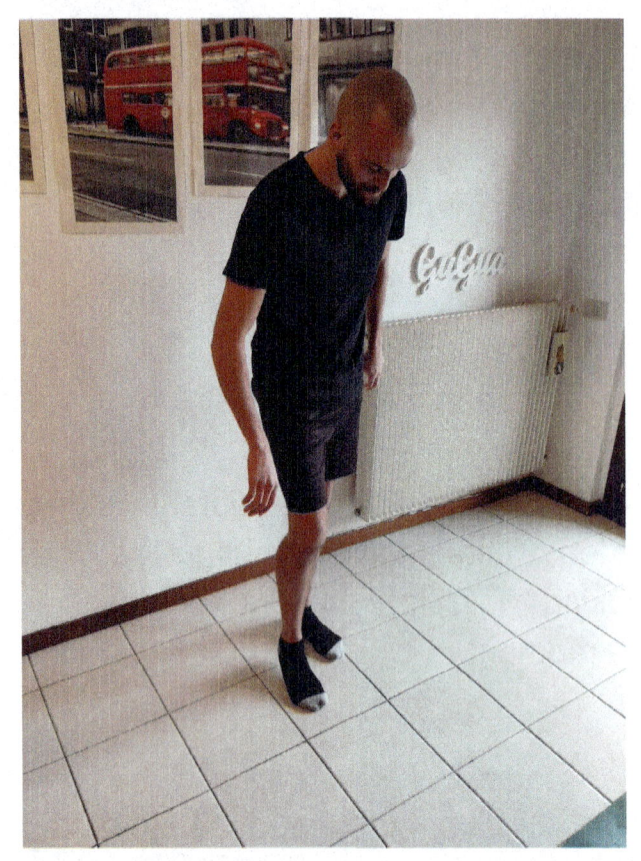

Step 1 - Run on the spot while shaking your arms.

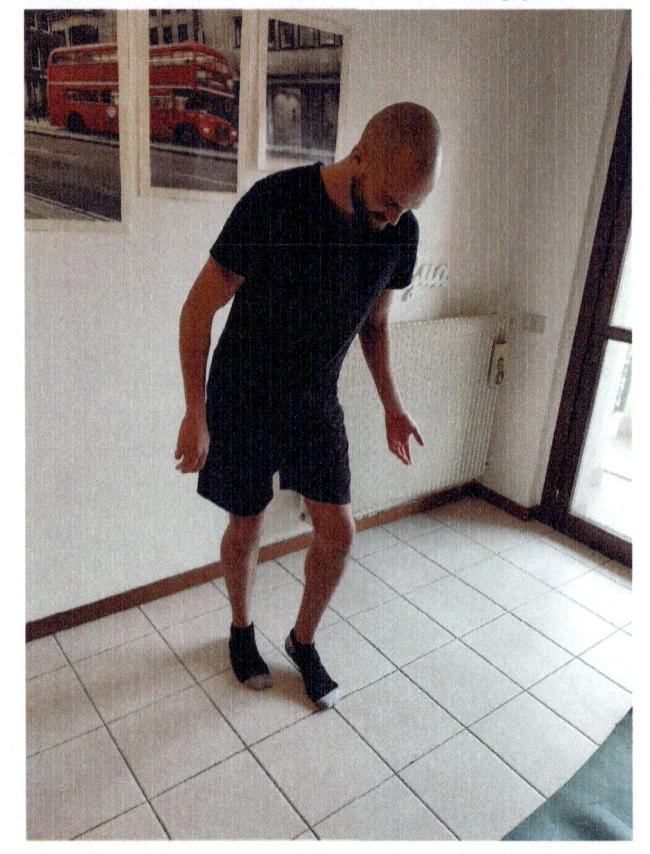

Step 2 - Keep repeating this movement for the mentioned seconds.

How to do it:

- Start by standing with arms at your sides and feet slightly closer than shoulder-width apart.
- Jog on the spot and shake your arms, focusing on releasing all the muscle tension in your upper body—emphasize exhaling deeply as you do so.
- Continue for the mentioned duration in seconds.

Note:

A fantastic, gentle cardio exercise that certainly helps burn calories. Also, concentrate on shaking your upper body to release all the stress and anxiety within you. Being and feeling relaxed while doing this movement is crucial for its effectiveness.

STAND ROCK SIDE TO SIDE

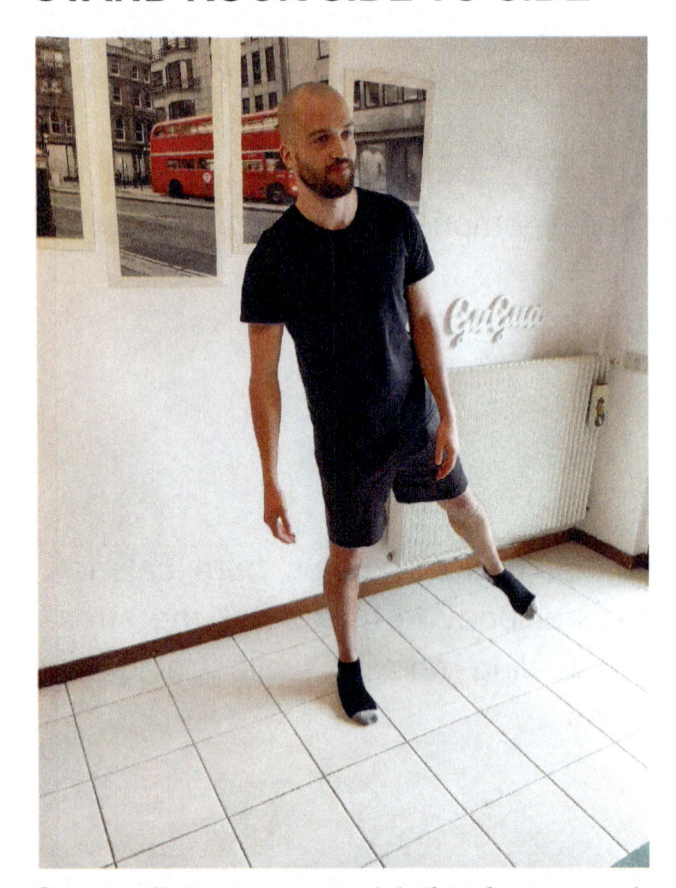

Step 1 - Balance on your right foot for a second.

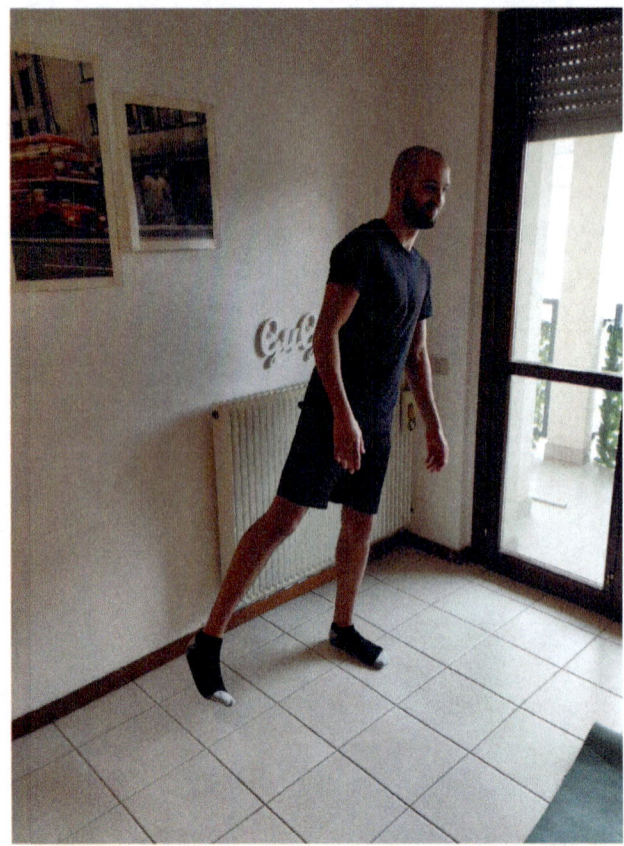

Step 2 - Then, bring your body on the left foot. Repeat the steps for the mentioned seconds.

How to do it:

- Start by standing with your feet slightly wider than hip-width apart, and arms at your sides.
- Then, step slightly to the side with your right foot and balance on it. Hold that position for 1 second.
- Lastly, repeat the movement on the other side, as shown in step 2.
- Keep alternating between these two movements for the mentioned seconds.

Note:

It is of vital importance to pay attention to your body as you do this. Focus on your feet to feel more balance (and spread your arms wide for further assistance if required). Keep breathing normally without interfering with it. For some people, it's normal to hold their breath, but avoid doing so for maximal effectiveness.

STAND ROCK BACK AND FORTH

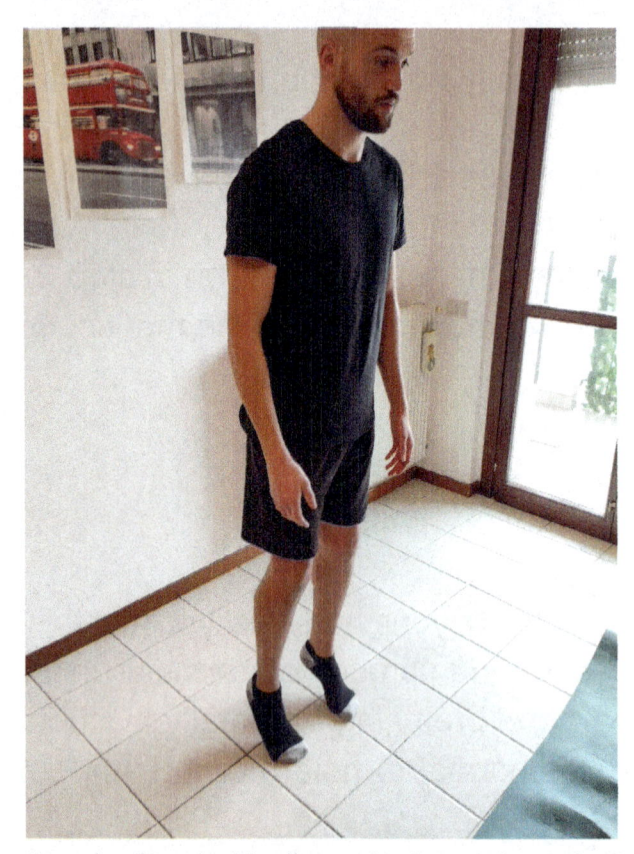

Step 1- Stand with all your body weight on the ball of your feet.

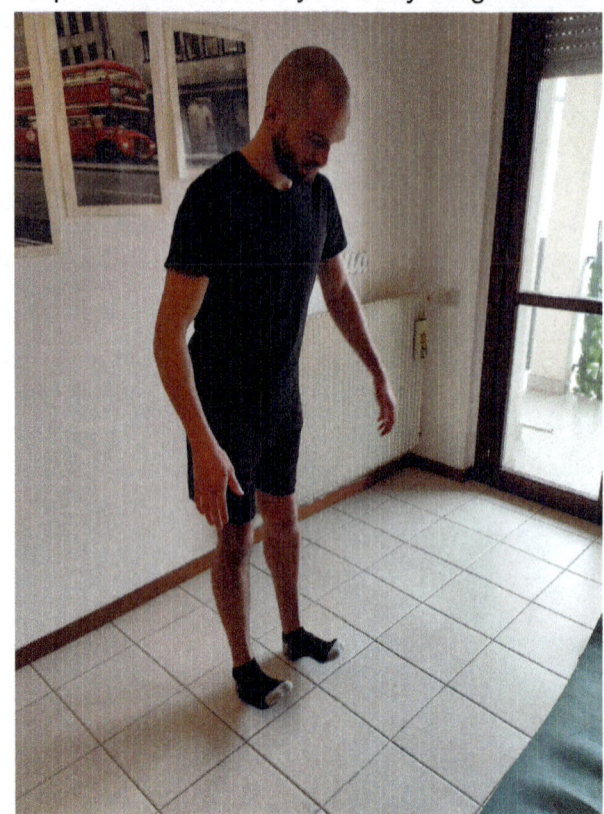

Step 2 - Rock backwards and stand on your heels. Keep repeating those two steps for the mentioned seconds.

How to do it:

- Stand and bring all your body weight onto the balls of your feet by lifting your heels.
- Then, rock backward and put all your body weight on your heels.
- Keep shifting the body weight from heels to toes for the mentioned duration. Pay attention to how your body feels as you do so.

Note:

If you feel a lack of balance, especially when balancing on your heels, do these two things:
1. Open up your arms to help with balance.
2. Hold that position for just a quick moment to reduce the chance of losing balance.

This is a great exercise to focus on your feet and feel how your body responds. Keep breathing without changing the breathing pattern.

FRONTAL RELEASE LUNGE

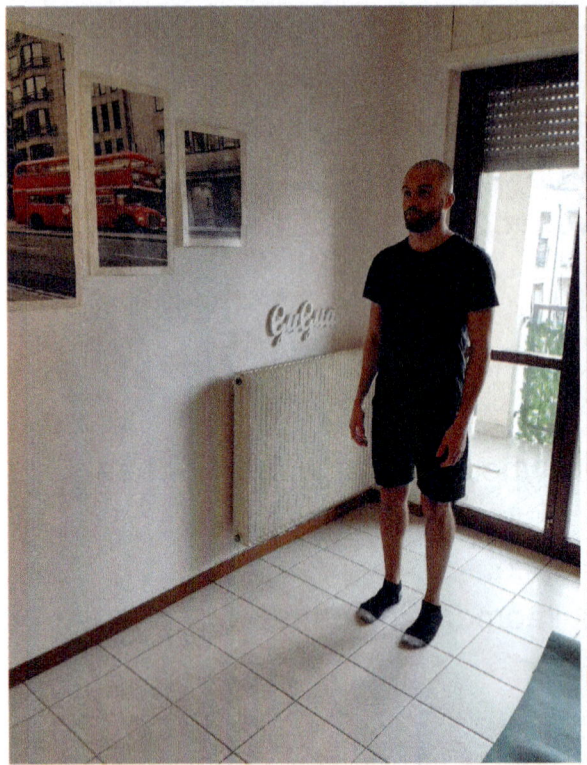

Step 1 - Stand with feet shoulder width apart and arms next to the body.

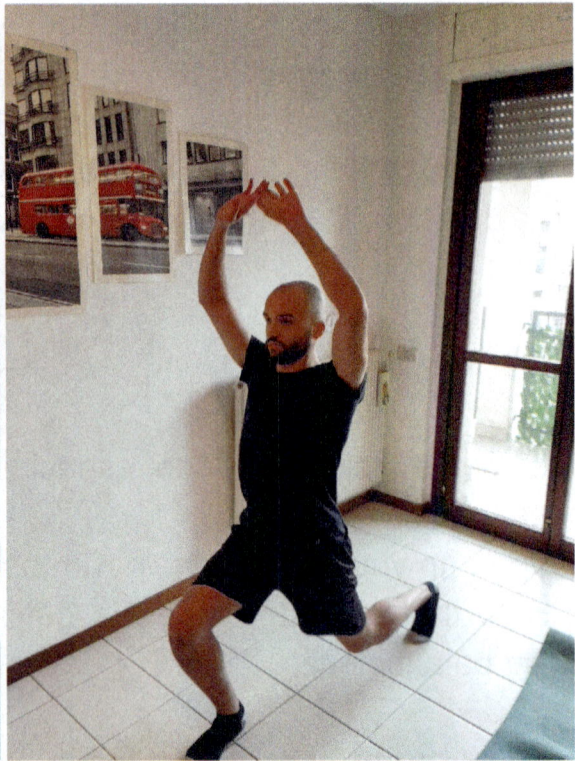

Step 2 - Lunge forward and reach over your head with your arms. Then, return to the starting position.

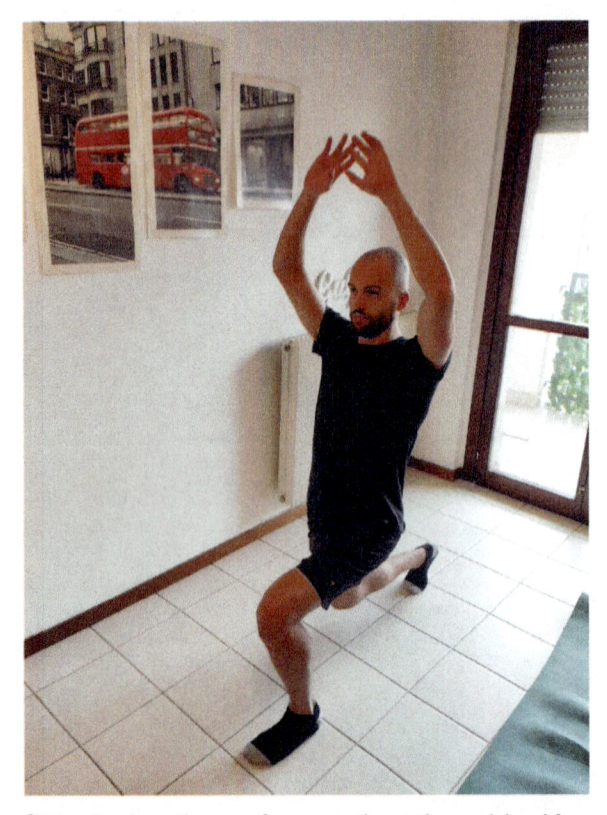

Step 3 - Lastly, perform to the other side. Keep alternating the sides for the mentioned reps.

How to do it:

- Stand with feet hip-width apart and arms at your sides.
- Then, lunge forward with your right leg (right thigh parallel to the floor and left knee almost touching the floor). Extend your arms as you do so and exhale.
- Come back to the starting position and repeat on the left side. Keep alternating sides for the mentioned number of repetitions.

Note:

If you lack balance, I would suggest you look at a specific point a few feet away. This will help you stabilize your body. Also, make sure to inhale as you come back to the starting position. Focus on releasing all the tension as you lunge and inhaling all the energy around you as you return to the starting position.

28-DAY PLAN

This 28-day plan is designed to improve your mental and physical well-being. A few minutes of focused physical activity each day can make a significant difference in your life. In order to achieve the best results, the daily workouts need to be followed strictly and repetitions should not be changed, except if you feel unwell.

Not only will you be able to improve your flexibility and strength, but you will also learn how to better manage stress and anxiety by participating in this programme. You will not only get a better understanding of your body and emotions. In addition to performing the movements, it is crucial to pay attention to your feelings and breathing as well.

This workout connects your body and mind by using basic breathing techniques to relax tension in your muscles and quiet your thoughts. During the workouts, focusing on your breath allows you to be more 'in the moment.'

Breathing and body awareness are key factors. This programme will not only make you feel better, but it will also make you look better.

Commonly shared feedback on the plan:

- **"I lost weight without even having to run"**
  These exercises burn calories and can be done in a small space, without the need for long runs or extensive workouts.

- **"Feeling more flexible and reduce back pain"**
  Flexibility is one of the areas that these exercises focus on. It will improve rapidly as the exercises require you to move in different ways, enhancing your full-body flexibility, which has many benefits.

- **"I feel energized"**
  Waking up every morning feeling recharged and looking forward to performing the workout is a great feeling to have.

- **"I feel less stressed"**
  The goal of the exercises is to relieve muscle tension, which is associated with stress. Additionally, the integrated breathing techniques naturally lower stress levels. Sustaining regularity will greatly improve your outcomes.

- **"I feel more happy and I feel more relaxed"**
  Somatic exercise makes you feel like yourself and calms your mind, which adds excitement to your life. You'll feel better and be less sensitive to stressful situations if you release tension and stress during your workouts.

DAY 1 - Repeat twice.

EXERCISE	REPETITIONS	PAGE NUMBER
KNEE GRAB SEATED	5 reps each side (alternated)	21
PUSH WALL	3 reps each side (alternated)	47
FLOATED CRAWLING	6 reps	9
LATERAL LUNGE AND REACH	5 reps each side (alternated)	35
SKIING	30 seconds	29
PIGEON POSE	3 reps each side (alternated)	43
SEATED WINDSHIELD WIPERS	5 reps	11

DAY 2 - Repeat twice.

EXERCISE	REPETITIONS	PAGE NUMBER
ROBOT	30 seconds	41
ROLLING PATTERN	4 reps each side (alternated)	13
STAND ROCK SIDE TO SIDE	30 seconds	53
SEATED WINDSHIELD WIPERS	5 reps each side (alternated)	11
PUSH OUT IN FRONT	10 reps	27
DOWNWARD DOG	4 reps	39
OPEN HEART	6 reps	17

DAY 3 - Repeat twice.

EXERCISE	REPETITIONS	PAGE NUMBER
SOMATIC HIP MOVEMENT	30 seconds	25
STOMP YOUR HEELS	60 seconds	49
SOMATIC SHAKING	30 seconds	31
RUN SHAKE	60 seconds	51
FLOATED CRAWLING	6 reps	9
ROBOT	30 seconds	41
HIP ROCKING ON STOMACH	60 seconds	33

DAY 4 - Repeat twice.

EXERCISE	REPETITIONS	PAGE NUMBER
LATERAL LUNGE AND REACH	5 reps each side (alternated)	35
BRUSHING BODY DOWN	6 reps	15
PIGEON POSE	4 reps each side (alternated)	43
FAWN	6 reps	37
BREATHING CIRCLE	5 reps	45
OPEN HEART	6 reps	17
SKIING	30 seconds	29

DAY 5 - Repeat twice.

EXERCISE	REPETITIONS	PAGE NUMBER
KNEE GRAB LYING	4 reps each side (alternated)	19
HIP ROCKING ON STOMACH	60 seconds	33
GROIN RELEASE	8 reps	23
FRONTAL RELEASE LUNGE	5 reps each side (alternated)	57
PUSH WALL	3 reps each side (alternated)	47
SOMATIC HIP MOVEMENT	30 seconds	25
STAND ROCK SIDE TO SIDE	30 seconds	53

DAY 6 - Repeat twice.

EXERCISE	REPETITIONS	PAGE NUMBER
PUSH OUT IN FRONT	10 reps	27
STAND ROCK BACK AND FORTH	30 seconds	55
KNEE GRAB SEATED	5 reps each side (alternated)	21
ROLLING PATTERN	4 reps each side (alternated)	13
BREATHING CIRCLE	5 reps	45
STOMP YOUR HEELS	60 seconds	49
SOMATIC SHAKING	30 seconds	31
RUN SHAKE	60 seconds	51

DAY 7 - Repeat only once.

EXERCISE	REPETITIONS	PAGE NUMBER
KNEE GRAB SEATED	5 reps each side (alternated)	21
PUSH WALL	3 reps each side (alternated)	47
FLOATED CRAWLING	6 reps	9
LATERAL LUNGE AND REACH	5 reps each side (alternated)	35
SKIING	30 seconds	29
PIGEON POSE	3 reps each side (alternated)	43
SEATED WINDSHIELD WIPERS	5 reps	11

DAY 8 - Repeat three times.

EXERCISE	REPETITIONS	PAGE NUMBER
ROBOT	30 seconds	41
ROLLING PATTERN	5 reps each side (alternated)	13
STAND ROCK SIDE TO SIDE	30 seconds	53
SEATED WINDSHIELD WIPERS	6 reps each side (alternated)	11
PUSH OUT IN FRONT	10 reps	27
DOWNWARD DOG	4 reps	39
OPEN HEART	6 reps	17

DAY 9 - Repeat three times.

EXERCISE	REPETITIONS	PAGE NUMBER
SOMATIC HIP MOVEMENT	30 seconds	25
STOMP YOUR HEELS	60 seconds	49
SOMATIC SHAKING	60 seconds	31
RUN SHAKE	90 seconds	51
FLOATED CRAWLING	6 reps	9
ROBOT	30 seconds	41
HIP ROCKING ON STOMACH	60 seconds	33

DAY 10 - Repeat three times.

EXERCISE	REPETITIONS	PAGE NUMBER
LATERAL LUNGE AND REACH	5 reps each side (alternated)	35
BRUSHING BODY DOWN	6 reps	15
PIGEON POSE	4 reps each side (alternated)	43
FAWN	8 reps	37
BREATHING CIRCLE	6 reps	45
OPEN HEART	6 reps	17
SKIING	30 seconds	29

DAY 11 - Repeat three times.

EXERCISE	REPETITIONS	PAGE NUMBER
KNEE GRAB LYING	4 reps each side (alternated)	19
HIP ROCKING ON STOMACH	60 seconds	33
GROIN RELEASE	10 reps	23
FRONTAL RELEASE LUNGE	5 reps each side (alternated)	57
PUSH WALL	4 reps each side (alternated)	47
SOMATIC HIP MOVEMENT	30 seconds	25
STAND ROCK SIDE TO SIDE	30 seconds	53

DAY 12 - Repeat three times.

EXERCISE	REPETITIONS	PAGE NUMBER
PUSH OUT IN FRONT	12 reps	27
STAND ROCK BACK AND FORTH	30 seconds	55
KNEE GRAB SEATED	5 reps each side (alternated)	21
ROLLING PATTERN	4 reps each side (alternated)	13
BREATHING CIRCLE	5 reps	45
STOMP YOUR HEELS	60 seconds	49
SOMATIC SHAKING	60 seconds	31
RUN SHAKE	60 seconds	51

DAY 13 - Repeat three times.

EXERCISE	REPETITIONS	PAGE NUMBER
BRUSHING BODY DOWN	4 reps	15
DOWNWARD DOG	6 reps	39
STAND ROCK BACK AND FORTH	30 seconds	55
GROIN RELEASE	8 reps	23
FAWN	6 reps	37
FRONTAL RELEASE LUNGE	5 reps each side (alternated)	57
KNEE GRAB LYING	6 reps each side (alternated)	19

DAY 14 - Repeat only once.

EXERCISE	REPETITIONS	PAGE NUMBER
BRUSHING BODY DOWN	4 reps	15
DOWNWARD DOG	4 reps	39
STAND ROCK BACK AND FORTH	45 seconds	55
GROIN RELEASE	8 reps	23
FAWN	6 reps	37
FRONTAL RELEASE LUNGE	6 reps each side (alternated)	57
KNEE GRAB LYING	4 reps each side (alternated)	19

DAY 15 - Repeat three times.

EXERCISE	REPETITIONS	PAGE NUMBER
ROBOT	30 seconds	41
ROLLING PATTERN	5 reps each side (alternated)	13
STAND ROCK SIDE TO SIDE	30 seconds	53
SEATED WINDSHIELD WIPERS	6 reps each side (alternated)	11
PUSH OUT IN FRONT	10 reps	27
DOWNWARD DOG	4 reps	39
OPEN HEART	6 reps	17

DAY 16 - Repeat three times.

EXERCISE	REPETITIONS	PAGE NUMBER
SOMATIC HIP MOVEMENT	30 seconds	25
STOMP YOUR HEELS	60 seconds	49
SOMATIC SHAKING	60 seconds	31
RUN SHAKE	90 seconds	51
FLOATED CRAWLING	6 reps	9
ROBOT	30 seconds	41
HIP ROCKING ON STOMACH	60 seconds	33

DAY 17 - Repeat three times.

EXERCISE	REPETITIONS	PAGE NUMBER
LATERAL LUNGE AND REACH	5 reps each side (alternated)	35
BRUSHING BODY DOWN	6 reps	15
PIGEON POSE	4 reps each side (alternated)	43
FAWN	8 reps	37
BREATHING CIRCLE	6 reps	45
OPEN HEART	6 reps	17
SKIING	30 seconds	29

DAY 18 - Repeat three times.

EXERCISE	REPETITIONS	PAGE NUMBER
KNEE GRAB LYING	4 reps each side (alternated)	19
HIP ROCKING ON STOMACH	60 seconds	33
GROIN RELEASE	10 reps	23
FRONTAL RELEASE LUNGE	5 reps each side (alternated)	57
PUSH WALL	4 reps each side (alternated)	47
SOMATIC HIP MOVEMENT	40 seconds	25
STAND ROCK SIDE TO SIDE	30 seconds	53

DAY 19 - Repeat three times.

EXERCISE	REPETITIONS	PAGE NUMBER
PUSH OUT IN FRONT	12 reps	27
STAND ROCK BACK AND FORTH	30 seconds	55
KNEE GRAB SEATED	5 reps each side (alternated)	21
ROLLING PATTERN	5 reps each side (alternated)	13
BREATHING CIRCLE	5 reps	45
STOMP YOUR HEELS	75 seconds	49
SOMATIC SHAKING	60 seconds	31
RUN SHAKE	90 seconds	51

DAY 20 - Repeat three times.

EXERCISE	REPETITIONS	PAGE NUMBER
ROBOT	30 seconds	41
ROLLING PATTERN	5 reps each side (alternated)	13
STAND ROCK SIDE TO SIDE	30 seconds	53
SEATED WINDSHIELD WIPERS	6 reps each side (alternated)	11
PUSH OUT IN FRONT	10 reps	27
DOWNWARD DOG	6 reps	39
OPEN HEART	6 reps	17

DAY 21 - Repeat only once.

EXERCISE	REPETITIONS	PAGE NUMBER
SOMATIC HIP MOVEMENT	45 seconds	25
STOMP YOUR HEELS	60 seconds	49
SOMATIC SHAKING	60 seconds	31
RUN SHAKE	90 seconds	51
FLOATED CRAWLING	6 reps	9
ROBOT	30 seconds	41
HIP ROCKING ON STOMACH	60 seconds	33

DAY 22 - Repeat four times.

EXERCISE	REPETITIONS	PAGE NUMBER
LATERAL LUNGE AND REACH	8 reps each side (alternated)	35
BRUSHING BODY DOWN	6 reps	15
PIGEON POSE	4 reps each side (alternated)	43
FAWN	8 reps	37
BREATHING CIRCLE	6 reps	45
OPEN HEART	6 reps	17
SKIING	30 seconds	29

DAY 23 - Repeat four times.

EXERCISE	REPETITIONS	PAGE NUMBER
KNEE GRAB LYING	4 reps each side (alternated)	19
HIP ROCKING ON STOMACH	60 seconds	33
GROIN RELEASE	10 reps	23
FRONTAL RELEASE LUNGE	5 reps each side (alternated)	57
PUSH WALL	4 reps each side (alternated)	47
SOMATIC HIP MOVEMENT	60 seconds	25
STAND ROCK SIDE TO SIDE	30 seconds	53

DAY 24 - Repeat four times.

EXERCISE	REPETITIONS	PAGE NUMBER
PUSH OUT IN FRONT	12 reps	27
STAND ROCK BACK AND FORTH	30 seconds	55
KNEE GRAB SEATED	8 reps each side (alternated)	21
ROLLING PATTERN	5 reps each side (alternated)	13
BREATHING CIRCLE	5 reps	45
STOMP YOUR HEELS	75 seconds	49
SOMATIC SHAKING	60 seconds	31
RUN SHAKE	60 seconds	51

DAY 25 - Repeat four times.

EXERCISE	REPETITIONS	PAGE NUMBER
BRUSHING BODY DOWN	5 reps	15
DOWNWARD DOG	6 reps	39
STAND ROCK BACK AND FORTH	60 seconds	55
GROIN RELEASE	8 reps	23
FAWN	6 reps	37
FRONTAL RELEASE LUNGE	6 reps each side (alternated)	57
KNEE GRAB LYING	6 reps each side (alternated)	19

DAY 26 - Repeat four times.

EXERCISE	REPETITIONS	PAGE NUMBER
BRUSHING BODY DOWN	6 reps	15
DOWNWARD DOG	4 reps	39
STAND ROCK BACK AND FORTH	45 seconds	55
GROIN RELEASE	10 reps	23
FAWN	6 reps	37
FRONTAL RELEASE LUNGE	6 reps each side (alternated)	57
KNEE GRAB LYING	4 reps each side (alternated)	19

DAY 27 - Repeat four times.

EXERCISE	REPETITIONS	PAGE NUMBER
BRUSHING BODY DOWN	5 reps	15
DOWNWARD DOG	6 reps	39
STAND ROCK BACK AND FORTH	45 seconds	55
GROIN RELEASE	8 reps	23
FAWN	8 reps	37
FRONTAL RELEASE LUNGE	5 reps each side (alternated)	57
KNEE GRAB LYING	6 reps each side (alternated)	19

DAY 28 - Repeat only once.

EXERCISE	REPETITIONS	PAGE NUMBER
BRUSHING BODY DOWN	4 reps	15
DOWNWARD DOG	4 reps	39
STAND ROCK BACK AND FORTH	45 seconds	55
GROIN RELEASE	10 reps	23
FAWN	6 reps	37
FRONTAL RELEASE LUNGE	6 reps each side (alternated)	57
KNEE GRAB LYING	4 reps each side (alternated)	19

CONCLUSION

Well done! You've just concluded a 28-day plan of somatic yoga and their incredible benefits. These exercises are beneficial to both your body and your mind.

If you want to continue, feel free to do the plan once again increasing the reps (one or two reps for exercises or 10 seconds more, according to the type of movement, works well).

I hope that you've realized that these workouts are a lot more than moving your body. They help you lose weight (especially if associated with a good diet), reduce stress, feeling relaxed and more connected to yourself. If you stick with it and do the exercises on a regular basis, you will undoubtedly notice improvements.

As mentioned at the beginning of the book, **for any questions or doubts related to somatic training and exercises feel free to email me at mertoncoreyfitness@gmail.com** - Looking forward to hearing from you!

As a result of the exercises that you have been doing, I hope you will continue to feel strong and healthy in the future. Thank you for joining me on my quest for better health. Continue forward and push to be the very best that you can be!